Pediatrics e-MCQ

Test Reviews For

PEDIATRIC BOARD EXAMINATIONS

Case vignettes and data interpretation questions in the multiple choice format with comprehensive explanations covered in 18 chapters of pediatric topics.

A. C. ANILKUMAR, M.D.

Diplomate, American Board of Pediatrics in General Pediatrics

Diplomate, American Board of Psychiatry & Neurology with Special Qualification in Child Neurology

Clinical Adjunct Assistant Professor, Pediatrics

Temple University School of Medicine

Associate Pediatric Neurologist, Geisinger Medical Center,

Danville, Pennsylvania, USA

Pediatrics e-MCQ

This book is protected by intellectual property rights. No part of the book is to be copied, or reproduced in any form or disseminated to third parties without the expressed consent from the author and the publisher. Purchase of the print or electronic version of the book will give the buyer the expressed consent to use for professional academic purpose only

ISBN-13: 978-1480205307 (CreateSpace-Assigned)

ISBN-10: 1480205303

BISAC: Medical / Pediatrics

©2012 Sauparnika Publications

Pediatrics e-MCQ

Disclaimer

The purpose of this book is to highlight the associations and important features of many disease conditions. Care has been taken to verify the information presented as correct as possible at the time of the manuscript preparation.

Medicine is an ever changing science. The research and newer discoveries in the pathogenesis and treatment modalities always occur. The information contained in this publication should be taken in that context. The views expressed hence are not considered authoritative or meant to signify the standard of care in the decision making scenarios or medical conditions presented.

The drugs, devices or other therapeutic interventions mentioned in this book may or may not be FDA approved in the USA or similar regulatory bodies in various countries for the specific indication. Medical practitioners should follow the appropriate statutory guidelines in using the information provided, and have the responsibility of verifying the FDA status of these treatments and devices. They should refer to the monographs or package inserts published by the drug

Pediatrics e-MCQ

manufacturer for each drug or device. The authors or publishers are not responsible or may not be held liable for any errors, omissions or any consequences arising from the application of the information provided in this book. We hereby make no warranties expressed or implied in the treatment of any condition or in the accuracy, currency or completeness of the data contained in this book.

Pediatrics e-MCQ

Preface

This book is intended for the students in Pediatrics including residents in training and thousands of test takers of USMLE® and the American Board of Pediatrics Examination for the Certification in General Pediatrics. More than a self-assessment test, this book is designed as a concise reading material for anyone interested in the specialty of pediatrics.

The questions are organized in the format of different sub-specialty topics; but occasional overlapping has inevitably occurred. You will find the answers and the explanations in the last chapter. Multiple choice questions (MCQ) are created to test the ability to solve the problem in a time constrained manner. So if you try to improve your speed and accuracy, you will be rewarded in future testing situations. Explanations and critiques are given as concisely as possible to reduce the bulk of the book. You should always consult a textbook in Pediatrics if you would like to broaden your knowledge on the specifics mentioned.

In all the examinations, there will be a substantial amount of direct questions on factual knowledge, which the candidates will acquire while they are in training. I have tried to include as many of the real scenarios as possible, to challenge the problem solving skills of the candidates.

 Most of the questions are based on actual patient histories as they presented in my practice.

Pediatrics e-MCQ

In multiple choice questions, there will be more than one plausible answer for each; but one will be the correct answer expected. There will be few distracters, sometimes ridiculously impossible; you have to steer clear of them. A good MCQ will be the one which can distinguish candidates based on the knowledge and critical thinking. It should be devoid of ambiguities and grammatical traps.

I have tried to analyze the answers with a common sense approach. Rare things happen in the examination papers as well as in clinical pediatrics. If you find the problems presented in this book are useful, my effort is well rewarded.

I would appreciate your feedbacks on this publication, with constructive criticisms and suggestions, to help me improve the quality of the future editions.

Pediatrics e-MCQ

Dedication

To the memory of my late father,

Who taught me in school and guided me in life.

To my mother,

Who is the proudest person on my achievements.

To my wife,

For your love and support.

To my children,

Whose faces give me the spirit to stay in my practice.

To my patients and their guardians,

For teaching me more medicine than the books could.

To my teachers,

For the wisdom they shared with me.

To my students,

To make me realize that learning is a lifelong process.

A.C. Anilkumar

Pennsylvania, 2012

Pediatrics e-MCQ

List of Abbreviations

ADH	Anti diuretic hormone
ADHD	Attention deficit hyperactivity disorder
ALT	Alanine amino transferase
AST	Aspartate amino transferase
ATP	Adenosine triphosphate
BMP	Basic metabolic panel
BP	Blood pressure
BUN	Blood urea nitrogen
Ca	Calcium
CBC	Complete blood count
Cl	Chloride
cm	Centimeter
CMV	Cytomegalovirus
CO2	Carbon dioxide
CRP	C-reactive protein
CT	Computerized tomography

Pediatrics e-MCQ

dL	Deciliter
DMSA	Dimercapto succinic acid
EEG	Electro encephalogram
EKG	Electro cardiogram
EMG	Electromyography
EMS	Emergency medical services
EMT	Emergency medical technician
ESR	Erythrocyte sedimentation rate
F	Fahrenheit
FDA	Food and Drug Administration
FiO2	Fraction of Inspired Oxygen
FISH	Fluorescent in situ hybridization
FSH	Follicle stimulating hormone
G6PD	Glucose 6 phosphate dehydrogenase
H2	Histamine 2
Hb	Hemoglobin
Hct	Hematocrit
Hg	Mercury
HIV	Human immunodeficiency virus

Pediatrics e-MCQ

HVA	Homo vanillic acid
ICU	Intensive care unit
Ig	Immunoglobulin
IV	Intravenous
k	Kilo(thousand)
K	Potassium
L	Liters
LH	Luteinizing hormone
MCHC	Mean corpuscular hemoglobin concentration
MCV	Mean corpuscular volume
mEq	milli equivalent
Mg	Magnesium
mg	milligram
ml	milliliters
mm	millimeter
MRI	Magnetic resonance imaging
N.S	Normal saline
Na	Sodium
NICU	Neonatal intensive care unit

Pediatrics e-MCQ

O2	Oxygen
PCR	Polymerase chain reaction
PICU	Pediatric intensive care unit
PPHN	Persistent pulmonary hypertension
PT	Prothrombin time
PTT	Partial thromboplastin time
RAST	Radio allergosorbent assay
rbc	Red blood cells
RDW	Red cell distribution width
Rh	Rhesus
RNA	Ribo nucleic acid
RSV	Respiratory syncytial virus
SBE	Sub-acute bacterial endocarditis
SIADH	Syndrome of inappropriate anti diuretic hormone secretion
SLE	Systemic lupus erythematosus
SpO2	Oxygen saturation by pulse oxymetry
T3	Triiodothyronine
T4	Tetraiodothyroine
Tc	Technetium

Pediatrics e-MCQ

VMA	Vanillyl mandelic acid
vWF	von Willebrand factor
wbc	White blood cells
WIC	Women, infants, and children program

Pediatrics e-MCQ

Table of Contents

Disclaimer 3
Preface 5
Dedication 7
List of Abbreviations 8
1. Cardiology 15
2. Child Psychiatry 27
3. Emergency Medicine 34
4. Endocrinology 43
5. Gastroenterology 52
6. Genetics 64
7. Growth and Development 76
8. Hematology and Oncology 80
9. Immunology and Allergy 92
10. Infectious Diseases 99
11. Metabolic Disorders 116
12. Neonatology 120
13. Nephrology 131
14. Neurology 141
15. Nutrition and Fluid Management 155
16. Pediatric Surgery & orthopedics 160
17. Pulmonology 176

Pediatrics e-MCQ

18. Rheumatology 182
Critiques and Answers 188
   1. Cardiology 189
   2. Child Psychiatry 196
   3. Emergency Medicine 199
   4. Endocrinology 204
   5. Gastroenterology 208
   6. Genetics 213
   7. Growth and Development 219
   8. Hematology and Oncology 221
   9. Immunology & Allergy 226
   10. Infectious Diseases 234
   11. Metabolic Disorders 243
   12. Neonatology 245
   13. Nephrology 250
   14. Neurology 254
   15. Nutrition and Fluid Management 261
   16. Pediatric Surgery& orthopedics 263
   17. Pulmonology 270
   18. Rheumatology 273

Pediatrics e-MCQ

1. Cardiology

Pediatrics e-MCQ

Qn. 1

A three days old infant was brought to the emergency room with lethargy and poor feeding. The infant was born by an uncomplicated normal vaginal delivery and was breast fed. On physical examination, the infant was found to be afebrile, having a mottled skin and poor capillary refill. Systolic BP was 30 mms of Hg with a heart rate of 140 beats per minute. Chest showed equal air entry bilaterally with normal breath sounds, respiratory rate of 34. Heart sounds were soft with grade II/VI systolic murmur over the precordium. SpO2 was 82 percent in room air. Chest X-Ray revealed unremarkable findings. Blood glucose was 34 mg/dL. What is the most possible etiology of this infant's problem?

a) Diaphragmatic hernia

b) Hypoplastic left heart syndrome

c) Tetralogy of Fallot

d) Necrotizing entero colitis

e) Galactosemia

Pediatrics e-MCQ

Qn.2

A full term newborn developed respiratory distress soon after birth and was transferred to the neonatal intensive care unit. Physical examination was normal except for nasal flaring, rapid respiration and tachycardia of 262 beats per minute. Oxygen saturation was 90 percent in room air, which responded quickly to 35 percent of ambient oxygen. Core temperature was 37.6 degree Celsius. Infant has

a) Benign tachycardia, which will resolve within an hour

b) Symptomatic supra ventricular tachycardia needing treatment

c) Closure of Ductus Arteriosus

d) Ventricular fibrillation

e) Neonatal lupus

Qn.3

An infant born after 36 weeks of gestation is monitored in the NICU. The right hand pulse oxymeter reads 96 percent and right leg pulse oxymeter reads 90 percent in room air. When the infant cries, both readings become low. Infant was then placed in an oxyhood to treat hypoxia.

Pediatrics e-MCQ

Examination of the respiratory and cardio vascular systems was otherwise unremarkable. Chest radiograph showed clear lung fields and normal size heart.

What is your assessment?

a) Persistent pulmonary hypertension

b) Transposition of great arteries

c) Pulmonary sequestration

d) Congenital lobar emphysema

e) Transient tachypnea of newborn

Qn. 4

A newborn developed seizures and tetany on the second day of life. Serum calcium level was 6 mg/ dL. Physical examination revealed hypertelorism with anti mongoloid slant of eyes, short philtrum, mandibular hypoplasia, low set ears, and a systolic heart murmur on auscultation. What is the probable diagnosis?

a) Williams syndrome

b) Noonan syndrome

c) DiGeorge syndrome

d) Fetal alcohol syndrome

e) Marfan's syndrome

Qn.5

A two year old previously healthy child was admitted to the intensive care unit after being found having difficulty in breathing and having unresponsiveness. Mother reports a history of flu like illness for two days with decreased appetite. He was given over- the- counter children's antihistamine. On physical examination, lungs were clear to auscultation, muffled heart sounds with a rate of 110 and unrecordable blood pressure was found.

What is the probable etiology of child's problem?

a) Pneumonia

b) Myocarditis

c) Tetralogy of Fallot

d) Patent ductus arteriosus

e) Antihistamine effect

Pediatrics e-MCQ

Qn.6

An infant born to a mother who is receiving Lithium for Bipolar disorder was found to have a systolic murmur at birth. You are arranging an echocardiogram to rule out congenital heart disease. What is the most common cardiac issue with the use of Lithium in pregnancy ?

a) Coarctation of aorta

b) Patent ductus arteriosus

c) Endocardial cushion defect

d) Ebstein's anomaly

e) Congenital heart block

Qn.7

A newborn is found to have symptomatic bradycardia. EKG revealed second degree heart block. What is the significant maternal history associated with this condition?

a) Use of phenytoin during the pregnancy

b) Use of Bronchodilators during the pregnancy

c) Maternal history of SLE

Pediatrics e-MCQ

d) Maternal history of Amphetamine abuse

e) Maternal history of Diabetes

Qn. 8

A large for gestational age infant was born to a mother with gestational diabetes. Infant had respiratory distress and symptomatic hypoglycemia.

An echocardiogram will most probably show

a) Endo cardial cushion defect

b) Atrial septal defect

c) Ebstein's anomaly

d) Septal hypertrophy

e) Supra valvar aortic stenosis

Qn.9

A 12 year old child is seen in the clinic for a physical examination prior to attending a summer camp. He was previously healthy, with no history of chest pain, syncope or breathlessness on exertion. The last visit to physician was two years ago when he had an episode of acute sinusitis. There was no documentation of heart murmurs on that visit. Today you find a soft blowing systolic ejection murmur of grade II/VI at the left sternal border which changes intensity with posture without radiation. First and second heart sounds are heard normally. His blood pressure is on the 50th percentile for age.

What is your assessment?

a) The child has mitral valve prolapse and need further evaluation

b) This is due to a small ventricular septal defect which needs SBE prophylaxis

c) This is a functional murmur of no significance

d) This is due to patent ductus arteriosus

e) Child has valvar pulmonary stenosis

Qn. 10

A 16 year old adolescent was sent by his Dentist prior to a root canal treatment to clear him for the procedure. His mother told the dentist that he has a history of heart murmur. Mother is seeing a cardiologist for her mitral valve prolapse. On physical examination you notice a short systolic murmur at the apex and a mid-systolic click. You are going to advice that

a) He does not need antibiotic prophylaxis prior to dental procedure

b) He has mitral valve prolapse and needs antibiotic prophylaxis against endocarditis.

c) He should not undergo dental procedure unless cleared by the cardiologist

d) He should not get Lidocaine for local anesthesia

e) He has peripheral pulmonic stenosis, which is a benign condition

Qn.11

A six month old infant was found to have tachypnea and cyanosis after two days of probable viral upper respiratory tract infection. Physical examination revealed nasal flaring and chest retractions.

Pediatrics e-MCQ

Chest auscultation revealed normal breath sounds bilaterally, normal heart sounds and no murmurs. You order a portable chest x-ray which shows a large supra cardiac shadow with a normal heart shadow forming a "Snow Man" appearance. What is the most probable diagnosis?

a) Tetralogy of Fallot

b) Ebstein's Anomaly

c) Total Anomalous Pulmonary Venous Return

d) Transposition of Great Vessels

e) Pulmonary Embolism

Qn.12

Which of the following is associated with endocardial cushion defect?

a) Lithium

b) Phenytoin

c) DiGeorge Syndrome

d) Downs Syndrome

e) Turners Syndrome

Pediatrics e-MCQ

Qn.13

A nine year old girl is visiting for the first time for a school physical examination. She was apparently well prior to this according to her mother.

On examination, you notice a systolic murmur and split second heart sound. You obtain an EKG at your office. The EKG tracing shows normal sinus rhythm at 80 per minute with right ventricular hypertrophy, right ventricular conduction delay with rSR' pattern. There is right axis deviation.

What is your diagnosis?

a) Normal findings for age

b) Atrial septal defect primum type

c) Atrial septal defect secundum type

d) Persistent truncus arteriosus

e) Transposition of great vessels

Qn.14

A six month old child was admitted with respiratory distress and persistent cyanosis. He had a systolic murmur at the left sternal border and a parasternal heave. A chest x-ray showed boot shaped heart with clear lung markings. You diagnose this as a case of Tetralogy of Fallot.

Which of the following is not a part of this condition?

a) Right ventricular hypertrophy

b) Overriding dextropositioned aorta

c) Infundibular pulmonary stenosis

d) Ventricular septal defect

e) Patent ductus arteriosus

Qn. 15

Cyanosis is not the usual presenting feature in which of the following congenital heart lesions?

a) Tetralogy of Fallot

b) Tricuspid Atresia

c) Transposition of Great Vessels

d) Truncus Arteriosus

e) Coarctation of Aorta

Pediatrics e-MCQ

2. Child Psychiatry

Pediatrics e-MCQ

Qn.16

A mother brings her nine year old son to your office with history of increasing problems of hyperactivity at school and home. He was described as being "wired" and having difficulties with homework completion, staying in one place and delay in getting to sleep. You are planning to start him on stimulant medication. Which of the following medications will help him to get proper sleep?

a) Methyl phenidate

b) Amphetamines

c) Atamoxetine

d) Pimozide

e) Clonidine

Qn.17

A six year old boy with behavioral problems and asthma has been recently diagnosed as having ADHD by his psychiatrist. He was also found to be having signs of Tourrette's Syndrome.

Pediatrics e-MCQ

He was prescribed a long acting Methyl phenidate preparation.

What is the most probable side effect of the medication he will encounter?

a) Aggravation of tics

b) Weight gain

c) Aggravation of asthma

d) Seizures after albuterol treatment

e) Cardiac arrhythmias

Qn. 18

A seventeen year old was brought to the hospital with sudden onset of abnormal behavior at a park. He was combative, diaphoretic, and tachycardic with dilated pupils.

Which of the following drug ingestion is a possibility?

a) Phencyclidine

b) Cannabis

c) Heroin

d) Ecstasy

e) Cocaine

Qn.19

A nine year old was brought to the clinic for evaluation because of his academic under achievement. He constantly bullies other children in the school bus, initiates fights, deliberately destroys property, and has problems with homework assignments, reading and in written expression. He is not fidgety in the class, listens to some teachers, but has poor organizational skills.

Of the following diagnoses, the most probable one for this child is

a) Attention deficit disorder, hyperactive type

b) Attention deficit disorder, inattentive type

c) Attention deficit disorder, combined inattention/hyperactivity

d) Oppositional defiant behavior/ conduct disorder

e) Anxiety/ Depression

Qn.20

A child was diagnosed as having bipolar disorder and started on Lithium. She started to improve dramatically in her symptoms. Mother is anxious about the side effects of long term lithium use in this child. You are going to advise her that

a) Lithium can cause iron deficiency anemia and she should be on iron supplementation

b) Lithium can cause hypothyroidism and thyroid function tests should be done periodically.

c) Lithium causes hirsutism

d) Lithium can cause bone marrow suppression causing thrombocytopenia

e) Lithium can cause acute hepatocellular injury; hence Prothrombin time needs to be monitored.

Pediatrics e-MCQ

Qn.21

A sixteen year old girl is diagnosed as having Anorexia Nervosa. She has lost about 40 lbs of her body weight in 3 months. Which of the following complications is NOT associated with this condition?

a) Superior mesenteric artery syndrome

b) High Cortisol

c) Pancreatitis

d) Hypercalcemia

e) Cardiac failure

Qn.22

A three year old boy is brought for his annual physical examination. According to his mother, he had no delays in his development. But she describes him as, "Not very friendly." He repeats what ever he hears, but does not answer to your questions. He watches the same Thomas The Tank Engine video over and over, gets agitated when it is switched off. He does not have any siblings and does not like to share his toys with other children when they visit him. He frequently throws tantrums and bangs his head on the table.

Pediatrics e-MCQ

He had two febrile seizures during the last three months. EEG and MRI done in the past were normal. Urine metabolic screen was normal. You do not find any abnormalities in his physical examination apart from the abnormalities of behavior and speech

Your diagnosis is

a) Autistic spectrum disorder

b) Cerebral palsy

c) Attention deficit hyperactivity disorder

d) Normal development for a three year old

e) Social anxiety disorder

Pediatrics e-MCQ

3. Emergency Medicine

Pediatrics e-MCQ

Qn.23

A 2 year old child was brought to emergency room with history of ingestion of unknown quantity of prenatal iron multivitamin tablets from his mother's drug closet one hour ago. You are going to advice the mother that

a) There is no need to worry since only 4 pills are unaccounted for, in the bottle

b) Iron tablets will not cause any problems except transient stomach upset.

c) Child should have an X-ray of abdomen

d) Child should get immediate hemodialysis

e) Child should be immediately given Desferioxamine IV if serum iron level is more than 150mcg/dL

Qn.24

Emergency medical technicians brought a teenager found unconscious at the road side. His cervical spine is stabilized with a rigid collar. He is having jerking movements of eye lids and the corner of the mouth. Pupils are equal and reactive. He is breathing normally at 20 breaths per minute. No neurological deficit was found on examination.

You will

a) Remove the cervical collar because it serves no purpose for this patient

b) Obtain a toxicology screen

c) Give O2 via non rebreather mask

d) Give Lorazepam 5mg IV

e) Give a gastric lavage

Qn.25

A teenager was brought by her mother after she was found vomiting at home. She gave a history of taking "many" pills of Acetaminophen 500mg after an argument with her mother. Which of the following is a true statement?

a) She does not need any treatment because it was a gesture to gain attention.

b) She needs to have her Acetaminophen levels checked every 4 hours

Pediatrics e-MCQ

c) N acetyl cysteine is administered after 24 hours only if her AST level gets elevated.

d) Charcoal is ineffective in gastric decontamination

e) Charcoal and oral N acetyl cysteine should not be given simultaneously

Qn.26

A seven month old infant is brought to emergency room after seen swallowing a button cell (watch battery.) Parent tried to put hands in the child's mouth, but child did not spit the button cell out. You did a chest x-ray and found that there is a penny as well as a button cell inside the stomach.

Your plan is to

a) Reassure the parent that these foreign bodies will pass without problem

b) You call the gastroenterologist for endoscopic retrieval of foreign body

c) Give Ipecac syrup to induce vomiting

d) Admit the child to hospital till the coin and cell are passed in stools

e) Give sodium citrate solution to neutralize the alkali from the button cell

Pediatrics e-MCQ

Qn.27

A 4 days old infant was brought to emergency department with lethargy and cyanosis. Physical examination showed decreased capillary refill, unrecordable blood pressure and short systolic murmur. You started an intravenous line and gave a bolus of 20mL/ kg N Saline. The infant was placed on mechanical ventilation after tracheal intubation. Chest X-ray, CBC, serum electrolytes showed normal findings. Your next line of management is

a) Intravenous Adenosine rapidly

b) Intravenous Caffeine citrate

c) Intravenous Prostaglandin

d) Intravenous Digoxin

e) Intravenous Calcium gluconate

Qn.28

A previously healthy two year old child was brought by the mother with a history of lethargy and refusal of feeds for one day. Child was afebrile, without any respiratory difficulties. No vomiting, diarrhea or constipation was reported. Physical examination is unremarkable except few bluish Mongolian spots over the buttocks, mucoid rhinorrhea and inability to visualize the right fundus because of few retinal hemorrhages.

Your assessment is

a) Physical abuse

b) Coagulation disorder

c) Viral syndrome

d) Hypoglycemia

e) Meningitis

Qn.29

A Four month old infant was brought to the emergency room with seizures. There is no history of fever, cough, diarrhea or difficulty in breathing.

Physical examination showed no dehydration, rashes or any foci of infection.

CBC showed 14,000 wbc/cmm, 24% polymorphs, 65% lymphocytes, 4% eosinophils, 5% monocytes, and 2% basophils. Serum chemistry showed Glucose 61mg/dL, Na 128mEq, K 5.6 mEq, Cl 109 mEq, CO_2 21 mEq, BUN 19mg/dL Creatinine 0.4mg/dL.

What is the probable cause of hyponatremia in this child?

a) SIADH

b) Nephrotic syndrome

c) Nutritional: low sodium in the formula

d) Renal tubular acidosis

e) Diabetes Mellitus

Qn.30

You are examining an infant brought to emergency room on a Christmas Eve.

According to the mother, the child was found to be sleepy and anorexic for the last two days. She did not have any fever. Mother has severe headache and not feeling well and wondering whether "she is coming down with Flu."

Pediatrics e-MCQ

Physical examination does not reveal any abnormal findings. Pulse oxymetry revealed 99% saturation in room air. CBC, serum electrolytes, urinalysis were all normal.

You are going to

a) Discharge the infant with reassurance

b) Admit to the hospital for observation and notify the social worker

c) Order a CT scan of the abdomen

d) Order a carboxy hemoglobin level

e) Order a serum Ammonia level

Qn.31

A child is brought by EMS personnel to hospital after being accidentally submerged in a swimming pool at home. He was unresponsive and had apnea.

What is the commonest electrocardiographic rhythm seen in cases like this?

a) Atrial fibrillation

b) Atrial flutter

c) Ventricular tachycardia

d) Ventricular fibrillation

e) Asystole

Pediatrics e-MCQ

4. Endocrinology

Qn.32

A two weeks old infant was seen at the first well baby checkup. Mother reports that the child is vomiting a lot lately. This was not resolved by switching to soy formula, thickening formula with cereal and changing the feeding schedule. No other problems were noted by parents. This girl was born normally at term without any perinatal problems. The physical examination reveals a female infant without much positive findings except mild dehydration, prominent clitoris and deep pigmentation of vulva. Complete blood count shows normal results, serum chemistry revealed hyponatremia.

Your next plan is to

a) Order urine amino acids

b) Order serum ammonia levels

c) Order serum organic acid assay

d) Order urine keto steroids

e) Order urine metanephrines

Pediatrics e-MCQ

Qn.33

A 14 year old girl is seen in the clinic. Mother is concerned about the delay in menarche. Her sister, who is 12, attained menarche the year before. On physical examination, her height is less than 5th centile for the age. Breast development is in Tanner II, pubic hair Tanner II. She has body odor and few acne spots on the face.

Your plan is

a) Reassure the parent, wait and watch

b) Abdominal CT scan

c) Karyotyping

d) Vaginal ultrasound scan

e) FSH and LH levels

Qn.34

A 13 year old girl is seen in the clinic for concerns about a swelling of the thyroid gland. She does not have any intolerance to heat or cold. She denied any loss of weight, diarrhea, constipation, fatigue, menstrual problems. On your physical examination, you find the thyroid gland is uniformly enlarged and soft. There were no lymph nodes, bruits or tenderness.

What is your provisional diagnosis?

a) Colloid goiter

b) Hashimotos thyroiditis

c) Graves' disease

d) Follicular carcinoma of thyroid

e) Medullary carcinoma

Qn.35

You are examining a Russian immigrant adolescent in your office. The family moved out of Russia after they were evacuated because of the disaster in the nuclear power plant. You find few lymph nodes in the deep cervical area and some nodular irregularity of the thyroid gland. Child denied any history of loss of weight, intolerance to cold or heat, palpitation or fatigue.

Child's mother is concerned about the lymph nodes.

Your advice is that:

a) You are going to order a biopsy of the node and thyroid gland

b) The lymph nodes are so common in this age group and is benign

c) You will order an ultrasound scan of the thyroid gland

d) You will prescribe antibiotics for 10 days

e) You will get a CBC to rule out lymphoma because of the radiation exposure in early childhood

Qn.36

You have admitted an 11 year old boy with Diabetic ketoacidosis to the ICU. You start him on Normal saline IV, Insulin drip and monitor hourly glucose levels. You are adding Potassium chloride and Phosphate to the IV fluid. What is the rationale behind the supplementation of phosphate?

a) To prevent metastatic calcification because of the shift in ionization of calcium when the acidosis is corrected

b) To produce ATP in order to metabolize glucose effectively.

c) To replace the losses due to osmotic diuresis and to avoid acidosis due to excess chloride.

d) To prevent precipitation when sodium bicarbonate and potassium chloride are infused concurrently in the same IV line.

e) To facilitate the glucose and potassium transport in to the cells.

Qn.37

An obese boy was diagnosed to have Hyperinsulinemic dysmetabolic syndrome. What is the associated skin manifestation seen in these children with insulin resistance?

a) Spider angiomas

b) Erythema annulare

c) Acanthosis nigricans

d) Cavernous hemangioma

e) Heliotropic rash

Qn.38

A two week old infant presented with seizures and was found to have hyperinsulinemic hypoglycemia. Which of the

Pediatrics e-MCQ

following medications can be used as an adjunct in the treatment for refractory hypoglycemia?

a) Hydrochlorothiazide

b) Spironolactone

c) Diazoxide

d) Furosemide

e) Captopril

Qn.39

A two year old is brought to the emergency room with sweating, delirium and seizures. Initial finger stick blood glucose showed a value of 32 mg/dL. There is a family history of Insulin dependent Type II Diabetes in the mother. His mother is worried that the child is developing diabetes.

In order to pin point the child's problem, you are going to order

a) Insulin and Growth hormone levels

b) Cortisol and Growth hormone levels

c) Glucose tolerance test

d) Amylase and lipase levels

e) Insulin and C-Peptide levels

Qn.40

A 14 year old girl is visiting your office with complaints of severe acne. She has irregular scant menstrual periods for the last two years. On physical examination, she is very tall and obese, has hirsutism, pustulo nodular acne on the face, chest and back. Your diagnosis is

a) Poly cystic ovary syndrome

b) Hypothyroidism

c) Cushing's syndrome

d) Congenital adrenal hyperplasia

e) Turner syndrome

Qn.41

Which of the following is NOT an associated feature of auto immune poly glandular disease?

a) Hypoparathyroidism

b) Mucocutaneous Candidiasis

c) Pernicious anemia

d) Pheochromocytoma

e) Addison disease

Qn.42

A teenager is admitted to hospital following a head trauma sustained in a rave party. He is drowsy, but no evidence of focal neurological deficits. BMP showed Na 130 mEq, K 5 mEq/L, Cl 112mEq/L, CO_2 22 mEq/L, BUN 19 mg/dL, Creatinine 0.5 mg/dL Glucose 136mg/dL. Urine Na is 30mEq/L, urine specific gravity is 1.020

He is currently on IV dextrose normal saline.

What is the next step in the management?

a) Increase the intravenous fluids by 20% to treat the shock

b) Add Sodium bicarbonate to the IV fluids

c) Hyperventilate to keep the blood pH over 7.5

d) Restrict intravenous fluids

e) Change the IV fluid to 10% dextrose

Pediatrics e-MCQ

5. Gastroenterology

Qn.43

A mother is bringing her five month old infant to your office with history of diarrhea for three weeks. The child is fed mainly on regular cow's milk formula with rice cereals and mixed fruit baby food about twice daily. As the diarrhea worsened, she was asked to give oral rehydration solution by your colleague last week. The child has no vomiting. Stools are yellowish green, liquid consistency. Her peri- anal area is red and excoriated with bleeding points. A stool examination showed pH 5, positive for reducing substances, no ova or parasites, stool culture revealed no pathogenic flora

What is your diagnosis?

a) Viral gastro enteritis

b) Cow's milk protein allergy

c) Lactose intolerance

d) Early introduction of solids

e) Diarrhea due to oral rehydration solution

Pediatrics e-MCQ

Qn.44

A newborn develops jaundice at second day of life. He is otherwise doing well in the regular nursery. He was breast fed. Blood type is A Rh positive and mother's blood type is AB Rh positive. Serum bilirubin level is 8mg/dL with conjugated 4mg/dL

Which of the following causes could explain the infant's jaundice?

a) G6PD deficiency

b) ABO incompatibility

c) Hexokinase deficiency

d) Rh incompatibility

e) Alpha 1 antitrypsin deficiency

Qn. 45

Which of the following statements about lactose intolerance in children are true?

Pediatrics e-MCQ

a) Lactose intolerance is a congenital disorder

b) Galactosemia is associated with lactose intolerance

c) Stool pH in lactose intolerance is alkaline because of the loss of hydrogen ions in the stool

d) Lactose intolerance can occur after an infection with Giardia

e) Dermatitis herpetiformes is the skin condition associated with lactose intolerance

Qn. 46

Which of the following tests is considered to be most specific for Celiac disease (gluten sensitive enteropathy)?

a) Immuno reactive trypsin

b) Serum haptoglobulin

c) Anti-endomyseum antibodies

d) Anti-gliadin and anti-reticulin antibodies

e) Red cell Folate level

Pediatrics e-MCQ

Qn.47

High serum gastrin levels, gastric hyper secretion and Peptic ulcerations are commonly seen in:

a) Hypoparathyroidism

b) Systemic Mastocytosis

c) Atopic dermatitis

d) Celiac disease

e) Cystic Fibrosis

Qn.48

A one year old child was brought to the clinic by parents because of ongoing diarrhea for a month. He started having diarrhea and vomiting associated with low grade fever initially when his parents switched the cow's milk formula to regular cow's milk. A stool culture done initially did not grow any pathogenic bacteria. Stool tested negative for ova and parasites. Stools are watery yellowish, occurring four to five times a day. On physical examination, the child is active and in no distress. He is currently fed on oral rehydration solution and juices.

Most probable reason for the diarrhea in this child is:

a) Lactose intolerance

Pediatrics e-MCQ

b) Cow's milk protein allergy

c) Fruit juice consumption

d) Celiac disease

e) Intestinal lymphangiectasia

Qn. 49

A seventeen year old girl is visiting your office to establish you as her new Pediatrician. She was seen in different practices and emergency departments for her ongoing diarrhea and vomiting. She lost thirty pounds of her body weight during the last three months. She denied any loss of appetite and use of medications. She and her mother are really concerned about her weight loss. Vomiting happens in public places, and not in relation to food. Her stools are watery and without blood. In the last week, stool culture showed normal flora and no ova or parasites on microscopy. Physical examination revealed a thin anxious teen with unremarkable findings.

Your provisional diagnosis is:

a) Lactose intolerance

b) Irritable bowel syndrome

c) Crohn's disease

d) Anorexia nervosa

e) Bulimia

Qn. 50

A six month old is having diarrhea for one week. She had frothy yellow stools many times, intermittent vomiting and had lost about 3 pounds of her weight. She is afebrile. She is currently on regular formula and cereals. Parents searched in the Internet and thinking that she has Giardia lamblia infection. What is the most sensitive test for Giardia?

a) Stool microscopy for ova and parasites

b) Stool pH and reducing substances

c) Stool culture

d) Giardia antigen test on stool

e) Giardia specific antibodies in serum

Qn. 51

In children with duodenal ulcers

Which of the following is true?

a) Majority of them are not associated with H.pylori infection

b) C13 Urea breath test is sensitive and specific for H.pylori infection

c) Children do not normally develop IgG antibodies against H.pylori.

d) Proton pump inhibitors are contra indicated in children because of the interaction with growth hormone secretion

e) Barium upper GI series is very sensitive and it avoids the endoscopy in majority of symptomatic children.

Qn. 52

A four month old infant is admitted with multiple episodes of bradycardia and apnea lasting for up to two minutes after feeding. You suspect gastro esophageal reflux as the etiology

The most specific and sensitive test to confirm the diagnosis is:

a) Milk scan (Tc scintiscan)

b) Esophageal pH probe

c) Barium esophagogram

d) Response to H2 receptor treatment

e) Esophago gastro duodenoscopy

Pediatrics e-MCQ

Qn. 53

A five year old boy is brought to the office with history of frequent passage of small watery stools with fecal soiling started one week ago. Previously he had problems with constipation and had hard stools with rectal bleeding. According to his mother, constipation got resolved with the use of Senna laxatives. His diet is normal, with plenty of vegetables and fruit.

What is the etiology of his problem?

a) Hirschsprung's disease

b) Laxative induced diarrhea

c) Chronic constipation

d) Irritable bowel syndrome

e) Crohn's disease

Qn. 54

Which among the following treatments is not used for children with Crohn's disease?

a) Corticosteroids

Pediatrics e-MCQ

b) Tumor necrosis factor antagonist

c) Cyclosporine

d) 6 Mercaptopurine

e) Secretin

Qn. 55

A Child Psychiatrist requested your consultation on a 15 year old child with bipolar disorder and ADHD admitted to the hospital. He is currently taking Lithium and Methyl phenidate. He has poor oral intake and was started on IV fluids. His serum chemistry showed normal levels. Liver enzymes, Amylase, Lipase, coagulation tests were within normal limits. Viral hepatitis panel for A, B and C viral antigen antibody profile revealed normal findings. He had an elevated Bilirubin level of 5 mg/dL(unconjugated bilirubin 4.1mg/dL.) Urinalysis showed no bile salts or bile pigments.

What is your assessment of his problem?

a) Hepato cellular damage due to the medications

b) Chronic active hepatitis

c) Alpha 1 antitrypsin deficiency

d) Gilbert's Syndrome

Pediatrics e-MCQ

e) Drug induced cholestasis

Qn.56

A 9 month old infant developed gangrene of the small intestine secondary to intussusception. About twenty centimeters of terminal ileum was resected out. During the rounds on this patient, a medical student is asking you about the long term problems with this type of resection. Your probable answer is that:

a) He will develop chronic renal failure

b) He will have Iron deficiency

c) He will have Vitamin B12 deficiency

d) He will have Lymphoma of the small intestine

e) He will develop Rickets

Qn.57

A three month old infant was admitted with failure to thrive, intermittent diarrhea and anemia. Stools were semi solid or watery without blood. She was on soy based formula since birth. On further investigation, the child was found to be having hypo albuminemia. You suspect a protein losing enteropathy. Which is the best test to perform to confirm your diagnosis?

a) 24 hour Stool total protein content

b) Stool alpha 1 antitrypsin spot test

c) Small bowel biopsy

d) D-xylose absorption test

e) Breath hydrogen test

Qn. 58

A two month old infant presented with history of wheezing, eczematous skin rash and bloody stools. The child was breast fed with formula supplementation as needed. A stool culture showed no pathogenic organisms and microscopy for ova and parasites were negative. Stool pH was 6.5, no reducing substances were present.

What is the diagnosis?

a) Milk protein allergy

b) Pseudo membranous colitis

c) Necrotizing enterocolitis

d) Celiac disease

e) Crohn's disease

Pediatrics e-MCQ

6. Genetics

Pediatrics e-MCQ

Qn. 59

A six year old girl was seen in the clinic for follow up of her acute pyelonephritis. Her renal ultrasound scan was suggestive of horse-shoe kidney. On physical examination, she was found to have decreased femoral pulsations and a webbed neck. You will order further tests to rule out

a) Downs syndrome

b) Noonan syndrome

c) Williams syndrome

d) Turners Syndrome

e) DiGeorge syndrome

Qn. 60

You are examining a newborn after an emergency Caesarian delivery. He has wide epicanthal folds, small curved little fingers, flat occiput and a single palmar crease. You suspect a genetic syndrome most likely,

a) Fetal alcohol syndrome

b) Fetal hydantoin syndrome

c) Turners syndrome

d) Downs syndrome

e) Edwards syndrome

Qn. 61

A 6 year old child was seen in your office for concerns of obesity. When he was born, he weighed appropriate for the gestational age. He was seen in another pediatrician's office in the early infancy for failure to thrive. He was put on nutritional supplements. Now he is morbidly obese and mother says that she has to keep all the food locked up in the cupboard for fear that he will finish everything in a day. He was reported to be eating other children's food at school and he was not interested in academic pursuits, but only eating. On physical examination, you find a child with severe obesity, hypotonia and rudimentary genitalia. He had signs of developmental delay on screening.

What is your diagnosis?

a) Fragile X syndrome

b) Congenital hypothyroidism

c) Cushing syndrome

d) Prader-willi syndrome

e) Exogenous obesity

Pediatrics e-MCQ

Qn. 62

A child was seen in the neurology clinic because of developmental delay. You observe the child entering the room. She was laughing loud for no apparent reason with outstretched hands and has an ataxic gait. She has some dysmorphic features with mid face hypoplasia. Your preliminary assessment is that the child has

a) Asperger's syndrome

b) Angelman syndrome

c) Rubenstein-Taybi syndrome

c) Edwards syndrome

e) Lesch-Nyhan Syndrome

Qn. 63

Uniparental disomy is present when both chromosomes of a pair of chromosomes are inherited from a single parent. Genomic imprinting is seen when the phenotypic expression of the offspring depends on which parent the chromosome or genes originated. Classical example of imprinting is

Pediatrics e-MCQ

a) Turners syndrome and Noonan Syndrome

b) Marfan's syndrome and Homocystinuria

c) Angelman syndrome and Pradder-willi syndrome

d) Williams syndrome and DiGeorge syndrome

e) Cystic Fibrosis and Celiac Disease

Q. 64

A three year old with cerebral palsy and developmental delay is visiting the clinic. He was recently admitted to the hospital following an episode of acute pyelonephritis secondary to urolithiasis. He is currently on Cefuroxime by mouth. He was very uncooperative for being examined and bit his lips till it bled. He was hitting his head against the stroller in spite of his parent's attempts. You suspect

a) Alport's disease

b) Lesch-Nyhan syndrome

c) Tourette's syndrome

d) Asperger's Syndrome

e) Adverse effect of Cefuroxime Axetil

Pediatrics e-MCQ

Qn. 65

A 14 year old child was admitted to pediatric floor for treatment of spontaneous pneumothorax. He was tall and thin built, with no previous medical problems according to his mother. On physical examination, you notice wide pulse pressure and an early diastolic murmur. Your diagnosis is

a) Williams syndrome

b) Marfan's syndrome

c) Kartageners syndrome

d) Cornelia deLange syndrome

e) Noonan syndrome

Qn. 66

A 6 month old child is send to your clinic when the emergency room physician at the local hospital found hypercalcaemia on a serum biochemistry evaluation. Your physical examination revealed a child with no apparent distress, but having elfin-like facial features. There was an ejection systolic murmur heard at right sternal border, radiated to neck.

What is your diagnosis?

a) Williams Syndrome

b) DiGeorge Syndrome

c) Cornelia deLange Syndrome

d) Wolf Parkinson White Syndrome

e) Romano-Ward Syndrome

Qn.67

A 6 year old child was brought to your office for evaluation of academic underachievement. He was born normally to a 26 year old mother with no prenatal or perinatal problems. His developmental milestones were reported as "normal as any other kid" by the parent. On your physical examination you notice very prominent ears, tall and thin built boy who is having large testes. Your preliminary assessment is

a) Acromegaly

b) Fragile X Syndrome

c) Hypothyroidism

d) Precocious puberty

e) Pradder-Willi Syndrome

Pediatrics e-MCQ

Qn.68

An adolescent with gonadotrophin deficiency is diagnosed as having Kallmann Syndrome. Which of the following features is seen typically associated with this syndrome?

a) Heart block

b) Anosmia

c) Blindness

d) Cholestatic Jaundice

e) Renal calculi

Qn.69

An infant was born at 38 weeks of gestation. His weight was 2010 grams and noted to have dysmorphic features. He had microcephaly, short sternum, micrognathia, narrow hips and Rocker-bottom feet.

Your preliminary impression is that this child has

a) Edwards Syndrome (Trisomy 18)

b) Fetal Alcohol Syndrome

c) Fetal Cocaine Effect

d) Congenital Varicella Syndrome

e) Congenital Rubella Syndrome

Qn. 70

A tall adolescent was referred to you by his optometrist for evaluation of a genetic syndrome. He was found to be having inferiorly located lens on eye examination. He had scoliosis and pectus excavatum and pes planus.

Your provisional diagnosis is

a) Marfan's Syndrome

b) Homocystinuria

c) Waardenburg's syndrome

d) Galactosemia

e) Goldenhar Syndrome

Qn.71

A two year old child was seen for routine checkup. He had a fractured tibia last year and a clavicle fracture when he was 6 months. He was placed in foster care by the child protection agencies. Mother denied any history of short stature in the

Pediatrics e-MCQ

family. Mother has problems with hearing and poor dentition. Your initial concern about this child is that

a) Child will be prone to further abuse by the parent

b) Child has Achondroplasia

c) Child has Osteogenesis imperfecta

d) Child has Rickets

e) Child has Vitamin C deficiency

Pediatrics e-MCQ

Qn.72

Your order for a Fluorescent in-situ Hybridization (FISH) test for a child suspected for DiGeorge Syndrome is

a) FISH 22q11-

b) FISH 15q 11- 13

c) FISH 7q23-

d) FISH 20p12-

e) FISH 6p13-

Qn.73

A large for gestational age infant is born to a mother with normal prenatal history. The infant is found to have hypoglycemia, macroglossia, microcephaly and earlobe fissures. You suspect this as a case of Beckwith-Weidemann syndrome. In the future while following up this child, you will closely observe for the occurrence of

a) Cardiac failure

b) Tumors, including Wilms Tumor

c) Ataxia

d) Fractures of long bones

e) Diabetes insipidus

Pediatrics e-MCQ

7. Growth and Development

Pediatrics e-MCQ

Qn.74

A four year old boy is in your office for a routine well child physical examination. His past history is unremarkable for any medical problems. He can write his name correctly and say his first and last name. Which of the following ability is normally NOT expected at this age?

a) Identify and name four colors

b) Prepare cereal

c) Define what is an "Apple" and a "Fence"

d) Heel to toe walk

e) Copy a square

Qn.75

You are demonstrating a Moro response in a newborn to a group of medical students. Which of the following is NOT a true statement regarding this primitive reflex?

a) Moro reflex and Asymmetric tonic neck reflex are not seen in the same age group.

b) Unilateral or asymmetric moro reflex could be due to brachial neuropathy

Pediatrics e-MCQ

c) Unilateral or asymmetric moro reflex could be a sign of cerebral palsy

d) Persistence of moro reflex beyond 6 months is abnormal

e) Moro reflex involves extension, adduction and then abduction of upper extremity

Qn.76

A four year old is NOT normally able to draw which of the following shapes?

a) Square

b) Triangle

c) Circle

d) Cross

e) Smiley face

Qn.77

You watch a child in the waiting room of your office. She can make a bridge of three wooden cubes on the table. What is the least approximate developmental age of the child to do this task?

Pediatrics e-MCQ

a) Twenty four months

c) Thirty months

c) Thirty six months

d) Four years

e) Four and a half years

Qn.78

A child is seen in a behavioral clinic. She has microcephaly, mental retardation, stereotypical hand wringing movements, poor social interaction and defective language development.

Your diagnosis is

a) Autism

b) Asperger syndrome

c) Rett's syndrome

d) Angelman syndrome

e) Fragile x syndrome

Pediatrics e-MCQ

8. Hematology and Oncology

Pediatrics e-MCQ

Qn. 79

A 15 year old boy with Marfan syndrome is admitted with difficulty in walking and diffuse purple discoloration of the lumbar and lower thoracic area of acute onset. He had surgery for aortic valve 3 months ago and is on oral anticoagulation. Neurological examination revealed decreased pain sensation and diminished reflexes below umbilicus. Power was grade 2-3/5 in the lower limb muscles. Joint movements were intact.

Most probable diagnosis is

a) Aortic dissection

b) Post-operative thromboembolism

c) Anticoagulant induced hematoma compressing the nerve trunks

d) Multiple sclerosis

e) Malingering

Qn. 80

A five year old boy is suffering from epistaxis for one month. He did not have any history of allergic rhinitis or nasal symptoms. On questioning, mother said he had profuse bleeding at the time of circumcision. He had few dental extractions recently, which did not cause any abnormal bleeding. Mother has history of menorrhagia, but no history of epistaxis. His father died of some liver problems at the age of 45.

Coagulation profile revealed : PT -normal , PTT -prolonged , Bleeding time -normal, Fibrinogen - normal , Fibrin degradation products - normal, Factor VIII activity- decreased, vWF multimers -decreased .Your assessment is

a) von Willebrand disease

b) Hemophilia A

c) Disseminated intra vascular coagulation

d) Vitamin K deficiency

e) Liver disease

Qn. 81

A five year old girl is brought by parents to the emergency room when they noticed red spots with bruising on her body. She had some gum bleeding also. On physical examination, you notice widespread purpuric spots and petechial lesions. There was no lymphadenopathy or hepato splenomegaly. On questioning, parents said she had a upper respiratory infection one month ago with painful joints; but she is not taking any medications.

A complete blood count showed WBC 12,000/cmm, Hb 13.5g/dL, Hct. 37, Platelets 30,000/cmm. Differential count : Polymorphs 40%, Lymphocytes 50%, Monocytes 6% Eosinophils 3% Basophils 1%. No bands or immature forms. Your assessment is

a) Henoch Schonlein Purpura

b) Idiopathic(Immune)thrombocytopenic purpura

c) Acute Lymphoblastic leukemia

d) Allergic reaction

e) Systemic Lupus Erythematosus

Qn. 82

A 10 year old child who recently had an induction chemotherapy for acute lymphoblastic leukemia is presenting with runny nose and fever of 39 C to the emergency room. Her blood count showed WBC 1700/cmm, Hb 9g/dL, Hct 27, Platelets 170,000/cmm . Differential count Polymorphs 24%, Lymphocytes 63%, Bands 2%, Blasts 1% and Eosinophils 6%.

Pediatrics e-MCQ

What is your next step in the management?

a) Admit to the hospital for IV antibiotics because of neutropenia

b) Advice to take over the counter medication for the cold and follow up with her specialist as scheduled

c) Give oral Azithromycin for five days

d) Arrange immediate blood transfusion

e) Prescribe granulocyte colony stimulating factor as outpatient

Qn. 83

A 6 year old child with sickle cell disease is presenting with fever for two days. He does not have any bone or joint pain. Physical examination revealed splenomegaly of 10 cms from the left costal border otherwise unremarkable. Complete blood count showed WBC count 6,000/cmm, Hb 8g/dL, Hct 25, Platelets 78,000/cmm.

What is your assessment?

a) Parvo virus infection causing thrombocytopenia

b) Auto immune thrombocytopenia

c) Splenic sequestration crisis

d) Aplastic crisis

e) Infectious mono nucleosis

Qn. 84

A two year old child was found to be anemic on a routine WIC program visit. You are advised to evaluate the child as the child's pediatrician. Physical examination did not show any abnormalities.

The results of the blood tests are:

Total WBC 16,000/cmm Poly 33% lymph 60% Eosinophils 3% Basophils 1% Monocytes 3%, Hb 9.2g/dL, Hct. 29%, Platelets 210,000/cmm

MCV 73fL, MCHC 31g/% rbc, RDW 14, Iron 90 microgram/dL (normal 50-120), Total Iron binding capacity 300microgram/dL(normal 250-500), Ferritin 130ng/mL (normal 7-140)

Pediatrics e-MCQ

Hemoglobin Electrophoresis: Hb A 25%, Hb A2 30%, Hb C 0%, Hb F 10%, Hb S 35%. What is your diagnosis?

a) Iron deficiency anemia

b) Sickle cell trait

c) Thalassemia

d) Acute leukemia

e) Sickle Thalassemia

Qn. 85

A 14 year old girl is brought to your office by the foster parent. She is having a low grade fever intermittently for three days along with cough and difficulty breathing. No history of asthma or allergies in the past. On physical examination, she was found to be looking ill with congested nasal turbinates and throat. She had rubbery firm non tender lymphadenopathy along the neck.

Chest auscultation revealed occasional rhonchi on the right side. There were no other significant findings. You order a chest x-ray, which shows widened mediastinal shadow. Your provisional diagnosis is

a) Hodgkin's / Non-Hodgkin's lymphoma

b) Acute leukemia

c) Pulmonary embolism

d) Bronchogenic cyst

e) Pneumonia

Qn.86

A female infant born to parents from Greece developed jaundice on the second day of life. Total bilirubin was 9.2mg/dL, conjugated bilirubin 0.6mg/dL. She was feeding the formula very well and did not have any other problems. Blood type of infant and mother were O Rh positive.

Mother did not take any medications during pregnancy. She remembers that her physician had in the past advised her to avoid certain medications, but she does not know what the reason was. Your impression about the hyperbilirubinemia is

a) Caused by G6PD deficiency

b) Hexokinase deficiency

c) Neonatal hepatitis

d) Gilberts Syndrome

e) Hypothyroidism

Qn.87

You are on call for the pediatric floor including some patients from hematology oncology. The Intern working in the night is calling for advice on a patient recently started on chemotherapy. She is not having any fever or discomfort, but the Uric acid level is 9mg/dL and Serum Potassium is 6mEq/L.

You will advise the Intern

a) To continue with the regular orders because these are normal for patients on chemotherapy

b) Advice to start IV hydration, alkalinization and Allopurinol

c) To stop Chemotherapy

d) To obtain a renal ultrasound scan

e) To order a 24 hour urine creatinine level to check the renal function

Pediatrics e-MCQ

Qn.88

Mother of your patient is asking your advice regarding a recent diagnosis of Acute Intermittent porphyria in her husband. She wanted to test for the condition in the child.

You will order

a) Urinary porphobilinogen levels

b) Urinary coprobilinogen level

c) Fecal porphyrin level

d) Erythrocyte free protoporphyrin

e) Uroporphyrin levels

Qn.89

A three year old child was found to have a lump in his abdomen by his mother. She denied any history of constipation or vomiting or urinary symptoms. On physical examination, you notice a definite non tender firm spherical mass in the left para umbilical area. Urine VMA and HVA levels are normal. CT scan of abdomen revealed a homogenous 6 cm size cystic mass attached to the kidney on the left with involvement of inferior vena cava.

The probabilities are

a) Wilms tumor

b) Polycystic kidney

c) Neuroblastoma

d) Hydronephrosis

e) Phaeochromocytoma

Qn.90

A nine year old girl was admitted with fever of unknown origin. She had bilateral cervical lymph node enlargement without any obvious focus of infection. CBC showed thrombocytopenia and mild leukopenia. Serum Ferritin level was 6000. Bacterial cultures revealed no growth. EBV titers were normal. HIV antibody test was negative. Bone marrow aspiration revealed normal cellular marrow with many histiocytes.

Lymph node biopsy showed multinucleated giant cells.

The diagnosis is

a) Hodgkin Lymphoma

b) Hemochromatosis

c) Langerhans cell histiocytosis

d) Acute lymphoblastic leukemia

e) Non Hodgkin lymphoma

Qn. 91

A thirteen year old boy has been complaining of pain on the side of the chest. He denied any trauma. On physical examination, there was a diffuse tender swelling on the 5th rib on the right side in the midclavicular line. CBC showed normal findings. An x-ray of the chest revealed onion skinning pattern of bone destruction and soft tissue swelling next to the rib.

Most probable diagnosis here is

a) Osteomyelitis

b) Osteogenic sarcoma

c) Rhabdomyosarcoma

d) Ewing sarcoma

e) Benign bone cyst

Pediatrics e-MCQ

9. Immunology and Allergy

Pediatrics e-MCQ

Qn: 92

A Previously healthy two year old child is brought to the clinic with complaints of greenish nasal discharge for the last three weeks during the Winter, night time coughing and intermittent fever. Physical examination revealed well-nourished boy in no distress, bilateral effusion of middle ear, dark circles around the eyes, bilateral purulent nasal discharge, moderately enlarged tonsils and conducted upper airway sounds on lung auscultation. A complete blood count showed total WBC count of 16,000/cmm with 74% polymorphs, 10% lymphocytes and 10% eosinophils and 5% monocytes.

This child probably has

a) IgA deficiency

b) Kartagener's Syndrome

c) Allergic rhinitis with Sinusitis

d) A viral upper respiratory infection

e) A nasal foreign body

Qn. 93

Pediatrics e-MCQ

A four month old child is admitted to hospital for an episode of diarrhea which started one month ago. A complete blood count showed hypochromic anemia, but otherwise normal counts. Immunoglobulin assay showed Normal IgG, IgE and reduced IgA and an elevated IgM level. This child has

a) Severe combined immunodeficiency

b) X linked (Bruton) Agammaglobulinemia

c) Selective IgA deficiency

d) X linked immunodeficiency with Hyper IgM

e) IgG subclass deficiency

Qn. 94

Parents of a child recently diagnosed as a DiGeorge Syndrome is meeting you as their child's new Pediatrician. They are asking whether there is any treatment for his condition.

Pediatrics e-MCQ

your appropriate answer is that

a) Immune deficiency can be corrected by Thymic and bone marrow transplants

b) No treatment available other than periodic gamma globulin injections

c) Can be treated only before birth

d) Splenectomy is a useful treatment

e) Monthly human growth hormone injections are useful

Qn.95

A child is having recurrent sinusitis and pneumonia due to Klebsiella infection. Complete blood count showed normal findings . Immunoglobulin levels showed normal pattern . Sweat chloride is 10 mEq/L. Tetanus and diphtheria vaccine antibody titers are appropriate.

The diagnosis is:

a) Complement deficiency

b) Cystic fibrosis

c) Wiscott-Aldrich syndrome

d) Chronic granulomatous disease

e) Asplenia

Qn. 96

In continuation of the above case in Qn.4;

What is the best diagnostic test to confirm your diagnosis?

a) Flow Cytometry for CD11/CD18

b) Nitro blue tetrazolium test

c) Adenosine deaminase assay

d) Lymph node biopsy

e) Roebuck skin window

Qn. 97

A three month old infant is hospitalized for the treatment of skin ulcerations not responding to oral antibiotic therapy at home. His umbilical cord dehisced at the age of two months and had infection of the stump. This family was notified to child protection services by a day care worker recently.

Possible etiology of child's condition is:

a) Transient hypo gamma globulinemia of infancy

b) Leukocyte Adhesion deficiency

c) Child abuse

Pediatrics e-MCQ

d) Colonization with Group A streptococcus

e) Maternal Cocaine use during pregnancy

Qn.98

Flow cytometry to measure CD11/ CD 18 surface glycoproteins on neutrophils is useful in the diagnosis of:

a) Chediak-Higashi syndrome

b) Adenosine deaminase deficiency

c) Leukocyte adhesion deficiency

d) Complement deficiency

e) Chronic granulomatous disease

Qn. 99

A Child with a history of neurological disorder and lymphoma is admitted to the pediatric ICU with pneumonia. On physical examination, ocular telangiectasia was noted. Immunoglobulin levels showed absent IgA, low IgE and IgG levels.

The diagnosis is:

a) Severe combined immuno deficiency

b) Shwachman-Diamond syndrome

c) Myeloperoxidase deficiency

d) Ataxia Telangiectasia

e) Wiskott-Aldrich syndrome

Qn. 100

A 5 year old child with seasonal allergic rhinitis is seen in the clinic for acute maxillary sinusitis. He recently finished 10 days of Amoxicillin/Clavulanate for an ear infection. Today his ears show normally appearing tympanic membranes with minimal effusion. He is currently taking cetirizine 5 mg by mouth and fluticasone nasal spray once daily for last 3 months. His mother says he has trouble sleeping because of the nasal obstruction and cough.

What is the next best approach to the management of his problem?

a) RAST Testing

b) Skin testing for allergens and immunotherapy if needed

c) Add inhaled broncho dilator for use at night

d) Use a humidifier in his bed room

e) Refer for Polysomnogram(Sleep Study)

Pediatrics e-MCQ

10. Infectious Diseases

Pediatrics e-MCQ

Qn. 101

You are called to see a 9 months old infant in the emergency room, who is presenting with an intermittent fever and diaper rash started 4 days ago. On examination, child had conjunctival congestion, few small cervical lymph nodes, a desquamating rash on the diaper area and hands. A complete blood count showed WBC 7800/cmm, Hb 12 g/dL, Platelets 1023k, Differential count: Poly 54% Lymph 39% Mono 4% Eosin 2% Baso 1%.

Which of the following tests is to be ordered for this child?

a) Echocardiogram to rule out coronary aneurysms

b) Tc Bone scan to rule out osteomyelitis

c) Bone marrow biopsy

d) Antibodies to Borrelia burgdorferi

e) D M S A renal scan

Qn. 102

A five year old boy is seen in your office for fever, sore throat, abdominal pain and vomiting started the day before. On examination, his temperature 101.4F, respiratory rate 22, BP 100/70 mm. He has a faint red sand paper like rash on the sides of neck, cheeks, axilla and abdomen. He had petechial rash and erythema of the tonsils. The rest of the physical examination was unremarkable.

Your diagnosis is

a) Scarlet fever

b) Infectious mononucleosis

c) Influenza A

d) Lyme disease

e) Herpangina

Qn. 103

Which of the following is a notable cause of meningitis in newborns?

a) Pneumocystis carini

b) Listeria monocytogenes

c) Cryptococcus neoformans

d) Candida albicans

e) Borrelia burgdorferi

Qn. 104

You are discussing a case of acute otitis media to a group of medical students. Your list of common pathogens associated with otitis media includes the following EXCEPT

a) S.Pneumoniae

b) M.Catarralis

c) Non typeable H.influenzae

d) Viruses

e) Pseudomonas sp.

Qn. 105

You are talking to the parent of a 33 week gestational age preterm newborn in the nursery. You are discussing the vulnerability to infections like respiratory syncytial virus infection. Mother is asking whether there are any preventive measures against RSV.

Your advice is

a) Only contact precautions

b) Palivizumab injections monthly, during the RSV season

c) Ribavirin therapy

d) RSV immunoglobulin injection at discharge

e) Oseltamivir treatment at onset of RSV

Qn. 106

Which of the following antiviral agents are found to be effective against Influenza EXCEPT?

a) Oseltamivir

b) Amantadine

c) Rimantadine

d) Indinavir

e) Zanamivir

Pediatrics e-MCQ

Qn.107

A child develops fever, joint pain and malaise and was seen in the urgent care clinic. His physical examination is unremarkable except for the fever and a red circular rash on the torso. Parents denied any history of similar illness in the family or close contacts. He had traveled to Wisconsin last month to meet his grandparents who own a dairy farm.

Your provisional diagnosis is:

a) Rocky Mountain Spotted Fever

b) Lyme disease

c) Ehrlichiosis

d) Blastomycosis

e) Visceral larva migrans

Qn. 108

A three year old girl with no significant past illnesses was brought to the office with history of drooling, low grade fever for two days and refusal to eat. On physical examination, you notice multiple discrete circular ulcers with well-defined red margin and yellowish base distributed over the soft palate, buccal mucosa and tongue. You diagnose this as Herpangina

The causative organism of this infection is:

Pediatrics e-MCQ

a) Human herpes virus-6

b) Varicella zoster virus

c) Herpes simplex virus type 1

d) Ebstein Barr Virus

e) Coxsackie A virus

Qn. 109

An adolescent is seen in the office for lacerations on the back and neck after a cave exploration as part of his summer trip. He gives the history of scratches sustained after he was accidentally entered a cave, full of bats. He does not think he was bitten by them, but remembers having tough time getting two of them from his back and got scratched by them. He had a tetanus booster two years ago. You give wound care and advise him that

a) He needs Tetanus Toxoid injection

b) He should not be worried about Rabies because contrary to popular belief, bats do not transmit Rabies to humans.

c) He needs post exposure prophylaxis against Rabies

d) He needs Rabies vaccination only if dead bats are found in that area

e) He needs treatment only if he develops any signs of fever, malaise or neck stiffness

Qn.110

A one year old child developed failure to thrive, lymphadenopathy and recurrent pneumonias over three month period. You suspect HIV infection. HIV Enzyme immuno assay test is positive. Which of the following tests you order to determine the HIV disease activity in this child?

a) Viral RNA load

b) P 24 antigen test

c) CD4 count

d) HIV PCR

e) Western blot test

Qn.111

A parent is bringing her 6 year old son to you with history of fever for two days and pain at the side of neck. On physical examination, he was found to have tender lymphadenopathy in the right axilla and the cervical region. He has few abrasions on the shoulder which he admitted as due to a cat scratch.

What is the most probable cause of his illness?

a) Bartonella henselae

b) Pasturella multocida

c) Brucella melitensis

d) Mycobacterium canis

e) Babesia microti

Qn. 112

A two year old African American child was brought to your office with a tender circular oozing swelling on the occipital area noticed one week ago. Parent was applying Neosporin cream obtained over the counter and changed to hydrocortisone cream, without any obvious relief. There was hair loss around the lesion as well as few patches of alopecia on the temporal region.

Most effective treatment of this problem is

a) Oral Zinc supplementation

b) Psoralen with Ultra violet A light

c) Tacrolimus therapy

d) Griseofulvin

e) Oral Cephalosporin for ten days

Pediatrics e-MCQ

Qn.113

A 4 year old child was brought to the office after being bitten by her cat on her wrist. Her immunization status is up to date. You clean the wound and give a dressing with triple antibiotic ointment. You will also give

a) Oral Erythromycin

b) Oral Penicillin

c) Oral Amoxicillin & Clavulanate

d) Tetanus toxoid injection

e) Tetanus immuno globulin

Qn. 114

A college freshman is brought by parents for evaluation. He is having head ache, vomiting and low grade fever since he came home after partying with his friends during the weekend. He is irritable and does not cooperate to your examination very well. His physical examination shows temperature 102F pulse 96, BP 100/70 and respiratory rate 23. There is mild erythema of the pharynx and nasal mucosal congestion and photo phobia. Rest of the physical examination is negative except for his irritability and minimal stiffness of the neck.

Pediatrics e-MCQ

Your diagnosis is

a) Phencyclidine intoxication

b) Methamphetamine overdose

c) Acute gastritis due to alcohol binging

d) Volatile hydrocarbon inhalation

e) Bacterial meningitis

Qn. 115

A five month old infant was brought to you for evaluation. She had loose stools with blood started since the day before. She had a low grade fever, but no vomiting. She was otherwise doing well and had no dehydration. You ordered a stool culture and the laboratory staff called in later with a positive result of Campylobacter jejuni in the culture.

What is your plan for this child?

a) Start intravenous ceftriaxone

b) Start Amoxicillin

c) Start Erythromycin

d) Start oral metronidazole

e) No antibiotics

Qn. 116

You are administering Influenza vaccine to a child of fifteen years.

Which are the following is NOT a contraindication to the vaccine

a) History of Guillain Barre Syndrome

b) Tetralogy of Fallot

c) Allergy to Eggs

d) Anaphylaxis after MMR vaccination

e) Child with multiple sclerosis on high dose corticosteroids

Pediatrics e-MCQ

Qn.117

A five year old child is presented with fever and swelling of the parotid glands. There is mild tenderness on palpation of the gland.

Parotitis can be due to all of the following EXCEPT

a) Coxsackie virus

b) Mumps

c) HIV

d) Candida

e) S.aureus

Qn. 118

A seven year old child develops severe pain and discharge from the right ear after swimming in the pool. On examination at the office, the pinna was tender on movement and the external auditory canal is swollen and tender. Otoscope speculum could not be introduced in to the canal because of the pain and swelling. Yellowish pus was seen adherent to the erythematous canal.

The organism most often implicated in this type of infection is:

Pediatrics e-MCQ

a) S. pneumoniae

b) M.catarrhalis

c) H.influenzae

d) Pseudomonas

e) Klebsiella

Qn. 119

A child with sickle cell anemia is admitted with severe bone pain of the tibia. Bone scan showed increased uptake at the upper end. You suspect this osteomyelitis. Which is the most probable organism causing osteomyelitis in this child?

a) S.aureus

b) Salmonella

c) S.pneomoniae

d) H.influenzae

e) Klebsiella

Pediatrics e-MCQ

Qn. 120

A four year old boy is on treatment with steroid for nephrotic syndrome.

He develops fever, abdominal pain and vomiting. On examination, he has abdominal distension, guarding and rigidity. What is the diagnosis?

a) Acute appendicitis

b) Hydrops of gall bladder

c) Pneumococcal peritonitis

d) Renal vein thrombosis

e) Acute Nephritis

Qn. 121

An immigrant child was seen for the first time in the clinic after coming to the country the month before. He has an intermittent fever for many days, associated with profuse sweating. He has poor appetite and malaise. No cough, vomiting or diarrhea was reported. On physical examination, he was febrile, Normal findings except an enlarged firm spleen. No signs of meningeal irritation.

You are going to order

a) Chest CT scan

b) Thick and thin peripheral blood smear analysis

c) Lyme disease antibody titers

d) Immunoglobulin levels

e) Sickle prep

Qn.122

A teenager accompanied her parents to Asia on a missionary trip. One day, she visited a hospital for Leprosy (Hansen's Disease) patients and helped in the nursing unit as a part time volunteer. She is wondering how the leprosy bacilli commonly spread from one person to another. Your answer is

a) Spread by contact

b) Spread by nasal secretions

c) Spread by mosquitoes

d) Spread by blood transfusion

e) Vertical transmission

Qn. 123

A parent of your patient is going to Philippines for a two week holiday. Her child is now 8 year old and fully immunized according to the current regulations in the state of New York. She is asking about the need for any other immunizations prior to their trip.

Your advice is

a) The child should get Hepatitis A and Typhoid vaccination

b) The child should not need any more vaccinations

c) The child needs vaccinations only if the stay is more than two months

d) The child needs only malaria vaccination

e) Child needs only Cholera and Yellow fever vaccinations

Pediatrics e-MCQ

11. Metabolic Disorders

Pediatrics e-MCQ

Qn.124

A newborn infant is found to have seizures and hypoglycemia. Physical examination was unremarkable. Sepsis work up was normal. Serum cortisol, Insulin, growth hormone, lactate, and ammonia levels are normal. BMP showed hypoglycemia, but no acidosis. Serum bilirubin level is elevated. Urinalysis showed the presence of reducing substances.

Your diagnosis is

a) Glycogen storage disease

b) Galactosemia

c) Urea cycle disorder

d) Methyl malonic aciduria

e) Maple syrup urine disease

Qn. 125

Which of the following features is NOT a characteristic of the urea cycle disorders?

a) Developmental delay

b) Failure to thrive

c) Acidosis

d) Hyperammonemia

e) Coma

Qn. 126

Low levels of urinary ketones is seen in which of the following inborn errors of metabolism?

a) Amino acidurias

b) Glycogen storage disorders

c) Organic acidurias

d) Pyruvate dehydrogenase deficiency

e) Medium chain acyl coA dehydrogenase deficiency (Fatty acid oxidation)

Pediatrics e-MCQ

Qn.127

Homocystinuria is diagnosed in a child at seven years of age. Which of the following are the features possible in this child EXCEPT

a) Dislocation of the lens

b) Post-operative bleeding

c) Developmental delay

d) Cataract

e) Convulsions

Qn.128

A five year old child with developmental delay, dystonia and self-mutilating habits is diagnosed as having Lesch Nyhan syndrome. Which of the following is the chemical substance thought to cause the neurological damage in these children?

a) Guanine

b) Cystine

c) Hypoxanthine

d) Inosine

e) Uric acid

12. Neonatology

Qn.129

A twenty four hour old infant born to a Diabetic mother by normal uneventful vaginal delivery developed seizures involving right upper limb. She is otherwise asymptomatic. Blood glucose values are all over 60mg/dL. CBC showed WBC count 14,000 Hb 19g/dL, Hct 59, Platelets 240,000 /cmm. Serum electrolytes including calcium and magnesium are within normal limits. CSF obtained by spinal tap showed protein 30mg/dL, glucose 28mg/dL, WBC 5/cmm (3 lymphocytes and 2 monocytes) RBC 6/cmm

What is the most probable cause of the seizures in this infant?

a) Cerebral infarction

b) Bacterial meningitis

c) Insulin

d) Hypoglycemia

e) Intra ventricular hemorrhage

Pediatrics e-MCQ

Qn. 130

A thirty five year old mother of your patient is now 16 weeks pregnant. She is asking you about Alfa Feto Protein levels and its significance since she recently checked these things in the internet prior to her scheduled amniocentesis. Low alpha Feto Protein levels are seen in

a) Spina bifida

b) Anencephaly

c) Downs syndrome

d) Epidermolysis bullosa

e) Turners syndrome

Qn. 131

An infant was brought to the hospital after being born in the bathroom at the home of a teenage mother. EMS reports that the umbilical cord was tethered by the mother during the attempts to separate from the placenta. The infant was found cyanotic and limp. EMS personnel gave O2 via bag and mask for up to two minutes to establish the spontaneous breathing.

The possible complications are thefollowing EXCEPT

a) Polycythemia

b) Jaundice

c) Anemia

d) Sepsis

e) Hyperthermia

Qn. 132

Oligohydramnios is seen in

a) Tracheo esophageal fistula

b) Posterior urethral valves

c) Diaphragmatic hernia

d) Werdnig-Hoffman syndrome

e) Cystic adenomatoid malformation

Qn. 133

A 36 weeks gestational age preterm infant is reported to have vomiting and abdominal distension. She was on 24 cal/oz cow's milk based formula. Stools were tested positive for occult blood. Radiograph of the abdomen showed thickening of the bowel wall and air in the bile duct and bowel wall.

Pediatrics e-MCQ

Your diagnosis is

a) Necrotizing enterocolitis

b) Portal hypertension

c) Malrotation

d) Ileocecal intussusception

e) Clostridium botulinum infection

Qn. 134

You are called to attend an infant who was born after full term normal pregnancy and unremarkable delivery. According to the nurses, he developed having chest retractions and decreased oxygen saturations immediately after birth. They gave O2 via head box, but O2 saturations remained below 90%. Then they gave positive pressure ventilation with 100% O2 via Ambu bag.

 Instead of improvement, the infant deteriorated rapidly. You intubated the trachea and given the infant positive pressure ventilation. The color improved and the infant looked much better.

Pediatrics e-MCQ

What is the probable diagnosis?

a) Spontaneous pneumothorax

b) Diaphragmatic hernia

c) Patent ductus arteriosus

d) Transient tachypnea of newborn

e) Surfactant deficiency

Qn. 135

A newborn is found to have microcephaly, petechiae and thrombocytopenia. Ultrasound scan of brain showed periventricular calcifications. Child remained asymptomatic otherwise. Your diagnosis for this infant is

a) Congenital toxoplasmosis

b) Congenital Syphilis

c) Congenital Herpes

d) Congenital CMV

e) Congenital Rubella

Qn.136

An infant born to 37 year old mother by vaginal delivery was diagnosed to have Downs syndrome. Infant was asymptomatic. CBC done on the first day of life showed 40,000 wbc /cmm with 57% lymphocytes, 30% polymorphs,10% monocytes.

Your impression of the abnormal count is

a) Leukemoid reaction

b) Congenital leukemia

c) Neonatal sepsis

d) Laboratory error

e) Diamond Blackfan syndrome

Qn.137

An infant is born to mother with gestational diabetes. He weighed 4.3 kg. Infant had polycythemia and hypoglycemia. Which of the following complications are associated with diabetes EXCEPT

a) Ebstein anomaly

b) Renal vein thrombosis

c) Caudal regression syndrome

d) Short left colon

e) Hyperbilirubinemia

Qn.138

A preterm infant of 33 week gestation developed respiratory distress and was given Surfactant treatment. His respiratory distress improved initially, but after two days, he started to deteriorate. An echocardiogram revealed a patent ductus arteriosus. It was decided to close the PDA using Indomethacin.

The following are the contraindications for using indomethacin, EXCEPT

a) Necrotizing entero colitis

b) Gastro intestinal bleeding

c) Sepsis

d) Creatinine level more than 1.7mg/dL

e) Serum bilirubin more than 10mg/dL

Qn.139

A full term infant who was born to parents of Chinese descent, developed indirect hyperbilirubinemia within twenty four hours of life. There is no blood type incompatibility in the infant and the mother. Child was fed on regular formula and was otherwise asymptomatic. CBC showed normal findings.

The possible cause of hyperbilirubinemia is

a) G6PD deficiency

b) Hereditary spherocytosis

c) Pyruvate kinase deficiency

d) Alpha 1 antitrypsin deficiency

e) Neonatal hepatitis

Qn.140

Which are the causes of hyperglycemia in neonatal period EXCEPT

a) Infant of diabetic mother

b) Sepsis

c) Caffeine

d) Transient neonatal diabetes mellitus

e) Maternal steroid treatment

Qn.141

A two days old infant developed tremors, tachycardia and diarrhea. Urine drug screen was positive for cocaine.

Which of the following medications can be used in the treatment of drug withdrawal in this infant EXCEPT?

a) Chlorpromazine

b) Phenobarbital

c) Clonidine

d) Diazepam

e) Naloxone

Qn.142

An infant born by C-section developed blood in the stool within twenty four hours of birth. He was breast fed and was given vitamin K. Of the following tests, which one will help you to identify the origin of blood as maternal blood?

a) Kleihauer Betke test

b) Apt test

c) Guthrie test

d) Ham test

e) Allen test

Qn.143

A six hour old infant born to a diabetic mother developed seizures. There was no hypoglycemia. Serum electrolytes including calcium were normal. A brain ultrasound scan showed normal results. Which of the following is the most probable cause of seizures in this infant?

a) Pyridoxine withdrawal

b) Hypomagnesemia

c) Hypoxic ischemic encephalopathy

d) Septicemia

e) Polycythemia

Pediatrics e-MCQ

13. Nephrology

Pediatrics e-MCQ

Qn.144

A 10 year old girl presented with history of red spotty rash on the lower extremities, buttocks, calf and lateral thigh. She was doing apparently well prior to this except for a fever and gastro enteritis two weeks ago which resolved without treatment. Now she is afebrile, but has some pain in the right knee joint with minimal swelling. She has normal urine output and denied ingestion of any medication.

What is the probable condition?

a) Systemic lupus erythematosus

b) Post Streptococcal glomerulonephritis

c) Poly arteritis nodosa

d) Henoch Schonlein Purpura

e) Meningococcemia

Qn.145

A 3 years old child was admitted to Pediatric ICU with new onset seizures. Her past history is unremarkable. She was in Utah, visiting her grandparents and came back three days ago with some diarrhea and vomiting. She was given oral rehydration solution and Acetaminophen for the last two days at home. Her serum chemistry was showing Na 136mEq K 6mEq, Cl 110mEq/L, CO2 20 mEq/L, BUN 30 mg/dL, Creatinine 6mg/dL, Glucose 94 mg/dL. CBC showed WBC 9000/cmm, with 60% polymorphs, 30% lymphocytes 4% eosinophils and 5% monocytes and 1% basophils, Hb 10 g/dL Hct 31% Platelets 120,000/cmm. Peripheral smear showed few fragmented RBCs and Schistocytes.

What is the probable diagnosis:

a) Acute Nephritis

b) Hemolytic uremic syndrome

c) Campylobacter Gastro enteritis

d) Analgesic nephropathy

e) Electrolyte imbalance secondary to diarrhea

Pediatrics e-MCQ

Qn.146

A sixteen year old boy is presenting with bloody urine. He had an upper respiratory infection with sore throat a week ago from which he completely recovered. His urine output is normal and denies any fever or dysuria. He does not have any edema. His blood pressure is 110/78 mm. The most probable cause of hematuria is:

a) Post Streptococcal glomerulonephritis

b) Complement deficiency

c) IgA Nephropathy

d) Urinary tract infection

e) Nephrolithiasis

Qn. 147

5 year old girl of immigrant parents developed sudden onset generalized tonic clonic seizures. She had fever and cola colored urine for two days prior to this illness. On physical examination the child had bilateral pedal edema, healed pyoderma scars on the legs, temperature 38.5C, respirations 23 per minute, BP 146/110mms ,brisk deep tendon reflexes and otherwise normal neurological examination.

Pediatrics e-MCQ

What is your diagnosis?

a) Pyogenic brain abscess

b) Coarctation of Aorta

c) Dermatomyositis

d) Post Streptococcal glomerulonephritis

e) Systemic Lupus Erythematosis

Qn. 148

A male infant was born by C Section at 38 weeks of gestation for fetal distress. There was history of oligohydramnios. On the prenatal ultrasound scan, the infant had bilateral hydronephrosis. The infant's was passing urine by dribbling. There was no phimosis. What is the probable etiology of the problem?

a) Posterior urethral valve

b) Renal vein thrombosis

c) Congenital nephrosis

d) Diaphragmatic hernia

e) Fanconi Syndrome

Pediatrics e-MCQ

Qn. 149

A teenager was send to the emergency room when she was found to have a blood pressure of 160/110 mm in the office. She had a mild head ache for last few days, but no other medical problems in the past. Her urine output was normal. Apart from the elevated BP, the physical examination was unremarkable. Her complete blood count, ESR, Serum chemistry panel including BUN and creatinine were normal and Urinalysis showed normal findings. Urine VMA was normal. Plasma renin activity was elevated. Renal ultra sound scan showed no hydronephrosis or calculi, but the left kidney size measured about half the size of the right kidney

What is the etiology of the hypertension in this case?

a) Essential hypertension

b) Amphetamine abuse

c) Acute glomerulonephritis

c) Renal vein thrombosis

d) Renal scarring

e) Pheochromocytoma

Qn. 150

A three year old boy was brought to the office when the parents noticed the swelling of his scrotum, face and eyelids. He was doing well prior to this and denied any change in urinary volume or color. He did not have any fever. The physical examination revealed a happy toddler with generalized edema, but otherwise with normal features. Urine dipstick showed specific gravity 1.030, pH 6.5, Protein 3plus, nitrate, leukocyte, blood and glucose negative

What is the probable diagnosis?

a) Minimal change nephrotic syndrome

b) Acute glomerulonephritis

c) Poison ivy reaction (Rhus dermatitis)

d) Renal tubular acidosis

e) Angioneurotic edema

Pediatrics e-MCQ

Qn. 151

A preterm newborn is receiving total parenteral nutrition after a bowel surgery for necrotizing enterocolitis. He is on Cefotaxime, Vancomycin and Amphotericin B for sepsis. A serum chemistry showed Sodium 135 mEq/L, Potassium 3.2 mEq/L, chloride 110 mEq/L, BUN 20 mg/dL, creatinine 0.6 mg/dL

What is the probable etiology of hypokalemia?

a) Urosepsis

b) Vancomycin therapy

c) Amphotericin therapy

d) Lipids in the Total Parenteral Nutrition

e) Ileal resection

Qn. 152

A nine month old infant was admitted to hospital with a diagnosis of acute gastro enteritis and dehydration. She improved her oral intake and the intra venous fluids stopped. She started having more formed stools. A repeat serum

Pediatrics e-MCQ

chemistry panel on the anticipated discharge day showed Na 136mEq/L, K 4.4 mEq/L, Cl 113 mEq/L, CO2 11 mEq/L BUN 23 mg/dL, Creatinine 0.5 mg/dL. Urinalysis showed specific gravity 1.010, pH 6, and negative for glucose, protein, blood and WBC.

What is the probable diagnosis?

a) Hemolytic uremic syndrome

b) Acute renal failure

c) Inadequate intravenous fluid volume administration

d) Acute viral gastroenteritis

e) Renal tubular acidosis (distal type)

Qn.153

A three year old girl is undergoing evaluation of the urinary tract after a hospitalization for acute pyelonephritis. A kidney ultrasound scan showed mild bilateral hydro nephrosis. A voiding cysto urethrography revealed grade II vesico urethral reflux on the right side. A Technetium renogram showed the right kidney function as 60% and the left kidney function as 40% with reduced drainage from the left kidney.

What is the probable Diagnosis?

a) Vesico ureteric reflux with left uretero pelvic junction obstruction

b) Posterior urethral valve

c) Usual findings after acute pyelonephritis

d) Right side vesico ureteric reflux with nephropathy

e) End stage renal disease

Pediatrics e-MCQ

14. Neurology

Pediatrics e-MCQ

Qn.154

A six year old child was brought by parents when they noticed the child having seizures in the early morning. According to the parents he was healthy previously, no history of developmental delay or history of similar episodes. He did not have any fever or other problems. On examination approximately 30 minutes after the episode, the child was afebrile, awake and having a normal neurological examination. His CBC was unremarkable except for a slightly raised WBC count without significant increase in band forms. Serum chemistry including electrolytes, calcium and magnesium was normal. An EEG performed later showed Centro temporal spikes.

Your diagnosis is

a) Juvenile myoclonic epilepsy

b) Atypical febrile seizures

c) Absence seizures

d) Benign Rolandic epilepsy

e) Central pontine myelinolysis

Qn. 155

A teenager was brought with a history of seizures occurred at school. There was no history of trauma or aura prior to the episode. The seizures were generalized tonic clonic, lasting up to 8 minutes. The child was awake when you examined her. Her neurological examination was unremarkable except that you notice slight speech impediment and she could not give you a good history of her past illnesses. When you ask the parents, they tell you that she is in regular class with no history of learning disability or developmental delay. You ordered a urine drug screen, serum chemistry panel, and CBC, the results were normal. EEG and a MRI scan are scheduled to be done later.

What is your impression of this child's problem?

a) Cerebral infarction

b) Methamphetamine use

c) Herpes simplex encephalitis

d) Landau-Kleffner Syndrome

e) Mesial temporal sclerosis

Pediatrics e-MCQ

Qn.156

A three year old is admitted to hospital for treatment of acute gastro enteritis and dehydration. The child was previously healthy, with normal development and is fully immunized. Serum chemistry panel was normal. He received intravenous Dextrose with 33% Na Cl for one day. Stool culture was positive for Campylobacter. The child developed sudden weakness of lower extremity with absent reflexes. No seizures or change in sensorium were noted.

What is your impression?

a) Central pontine myelinolysis due to rapid sodium administration

b) Hypokalemic paralysis

c) Paralytic Polio Myelitis

d) Transverse myelitis due to Campylobacter

e) Guillain- Barre Syndrome

Qn. 157

A child was seen in the clinic for behavior problems. He was very hyperactive in the class, with disrupting behavior and in attention. These symptoms, according to parents, began at Kindergarten stage. He was started on Methyl Phenidate 18 mg by his psychiatrist 6 months ago. Your examination reveals a well-nourished boy of seven years, with no apparent distress. He kept his head tilted while playing with his hand held video game. His neurological examination was unremarkable except for a slight ataxia on walking. His mother said he like to be a "clown".

What is your plan of management?

a) A change to higher dose of Methyl Phenidate

b) Change to Dextroamphetamine

c) Check Vitamin B12 level

d) Check his thyroid function

e) Check VMA and HVA of urine

Qn. 158

A four month old infant was brought to the clinic with concern on abnormal behavior. He was found to nodding off or dropping his head in upright position, extends his arms and flexes his waist. Initially the parents thought he was just being sleepy, but lately these are occurring after waking up.

Your advice is that

Pediatrics e-MCQ

a) This is Sandifer syndrome, due to gastro esophageal reflux

b) This is Infantile Myoclonic Epilepsy

c) This is Infantile Spasms, which usually respond to ACTH

d) This is a normal sleep pattern of infants of this age

e) This child has colic

Qn.159

You examine an infant in the clinic during a well child visit. You notice a shagreen patch on the body and explain to the parent that he needs to be investigated for Tuberous Sclerosis Complex. The mother is asking you about the type of seizures the child might develop in the future.

Your response is

a) Absence seizures

b) Infantile spasms

c) Rolandic Epilepsy with Centro temporal spikes

d) Myoclonic epilepsy

e) Temporal lobe seizures

Pediatrics e-MCQ

Qn. 160

A three year old child was brought for evaluation because he has problems in getting up from sitting position and a waddling gait. Mother explains that he pushes his hands on the floor to get to an erect position. He does not have any other delay in his development. On examination, he has intact tendon reflexes, good muscle bulk and tone of the lower limbs. You do not notice any sensory or motor deficits. Examination of the hips shows no clicks and full range of motion. Your advice to the parent is that

a) This is a normal variant of motor development

b) This is due to undiagnosed hip joint subluxation

c) Child has slipped femoral capital epiphysis

d) Child has features of Duchenne muscular dystrophy

e) Child has features of Dermatomyositis

Qn. 161

A 10 month old child was brought to the emergency room with new onset seizures. Child was seen in the pediatrician's office earlier during the day for a red rash on the face and torso. The pediatrician diagnosed Roseola and advised the parents to give Acetaminophen for fever control.

Pediatrics e-MCQ

Physical examination reveals a temperature of 103.4 F, a widespread blanching erythematous rash, mild congestion of the throat. Rest of the physical examination is unremarkable.

Your diagnosis is

a) Reye's syndrome

b) Febrile seizures

c) Meningitis due to Neisseria

d) Scarlet fever

e) Kawasaki syndrome

Qn. 162

A nine year old child was seen in the clinic with complaints of "day dreaming" and parent wanted to check for ADHD. While you are talking to the mother, you are observing the child who is attempting to inflate a latex glove, then stopping it and staring in to air motionless for about 15seconds. She blinks her eye few times and smiles at you afterwards.

You advice the parent that

a) You need to start her on anticonvulsant after obtaining an EEG

b) You will start her on stimulant medication if she has inattentive problems at school and home for past six months.

c) You advice that she does not need any work up or medication

d) She needs to be tested for latex allergy

e) She needs to see a child psychiatrist to check for depression

Qn.163

A newborn was seen in the nursery. You notice a flat Port Wine stain birthmark extending from the middle of the forehead to the outer aspect of his left eye.

Mother is asking whether this will cause any problems in the future.

Your answer is that

a) This is flame nevus or stork bite, which is common in infants

b) This is cavernous hemangioma, which can cause thrombocytopenia

c) This is strawberry hemangioma, which can involute sometimes spontaneously

d) This is Sturge Weber syndrome and can have neurological sequelae

e) This is incontinentia pigmenti, a lethal condition

Qn.164

A 4 year old boy who was healthy previously, is admitted to hospital with history of inability of keeping an erect posture. His problems started after getting up from sleep. Parents denied history of any trauma, fever, medications and seizures. On physical examination, he was alert and active. Neurological examination showed normal reflexes and no neurological deficits except cerebellar ataxia. CBC, Serum chemistry, liver function tests, drug toxicology screen, urine VMA, HVA, CSF studies, MRI of brain, EEG were reported as normal.

Most probable diagnosis is

a) Neuroblastoma

b) Acute cerebellar ataxia

c) Multiple sclerosis

d) Guillain Barre syndrome

e) Encephalitis

Qn.165

A 4 year old girl is brought by parents with concerns of repeated episodes of sudden crying while sleeping occurring almost every week. The episodes lasted up to 5 minutes, the child crying for no reason. She did not talk to parents and did not have any recollection of the incident. There was no tonic clonic activity reported. Child was hyperventilating and sweating during the episodes.

Your plan is to

a) Reassure parents that these are benign night terrors

b) Arrange a work up for GERD and Sandifer syndrome

c) Obtain an EEG to rule out seizure disorders

d) Get a CT scan of head to rule out medulloblastoma

e) Get a 24 hour Holter tracing to rule out arrhythmia

Qn.166

A 10 year old girl is seen in the neurology clinic. She was sent by her family doctor with suspicion of a neurological disorder. Child developed sudden inability to open her eyes and difficulty in talking and swallowing. She can walk with assistance. She does not have any fever, cough, diarrhea, incontinence or constipation. She is not on any medication. On examination, the child is alert, not in distress. Partial pseudo ptosis was seen bilaterally. No wrinkles were noted on the forehead when she was asked to look up. Eyes can be opened forcibly. Pupils reacted normally. No facial asymmetry or other cranial nerve involvement. Deep tendon reflexes were preserved, normal power and tone of all muscles.

Your plan is to

a) Get an Edrophonium test

b) Get an EMG

c) Get a MRI of brain

d) Get Lead level

e) Get a psychiatric evaluation

Pediatrics e-MCQ

Qn.167

A 6 month old was coming for well child examination. The family moved from another state because of his parent's transfer. Child was doing well according to the parent. His height and weight were on the 75th percentile and head circumference on the 5th percentile. There is ridging on the sutures. Anterior fontanel is closed. Child's motor, adaptive and language skills are normal for age. Muscle tone is normal. No neurological deficit found. His eyes are down-turned. Rest of the examination was normal

Your diagnosis is

a) Cranio synostosis

b) Normal development

c) Hyperthyroidism

d) Downs syndrome

e) Dandy walker malformation

Qn.168

You are examining a full term, large for gestation, newborn infant in the nursery. Mother had gestational diabetes, but no other problems during the delivery except a shoulder dystocia and prolonged second stage.

On examination, you find an incomplete moro reflex with reduced shoulder movements on the right side, no evidence of hypotonia, movements of joints are within normal range. No tenderness, crepitus or clicks elicited on the bones or joints.

What is your diagnosis?

a) Periventricular leukomalacia

b) Insulin embryopathy

c) Brachial neuropathy

d) Cerebral infarction

e) Fractured clavicle

15. Nutrition and Fluid Management

Pediatrics e-MCQ

Qn.169

A breast fed 4 month old African American infant is seen in the well baby clinic. On examination, the anterior fontanel was large, flattened skull and prominent costochondral junctions with a subcostal sulcus was found. Which of the following findings will be seen in a blood test of this infant?

a) Elevated Calcium

b) Elevated Phosphorous

c) Elevated alkaline phosphatase

d) Elevated serum 25-hydroxy cholecalciferol

e) Elevated serum Iron

Qn. 170

A teenager who is on nutritional supplements is complaining of constant head ache. All the work-ups done including MRI of the brain were negative. Finally, a diagnosis of benign intra cranial hypertension was made and he underwent a lumbar puncture. The headache got resolved after the lumbar puncture and he decided to stop the nutritional supplementation.

Pediatrics e-MCQ

Which of the following nutrients probably caused his head ache?

a) Vitamin A

b) Vitamin B complex

c) Vitamin C

d) Vitamin D

e) Vitamin E

Qn. 171

A new born developed myoclonic seizures and startle response on the third day of life after an uneventful normal birth at term. Full sepsis work up, BMP, Cultures, MRI of the brain, urine toxicology screens were negative.

What prenatal history you will specifically obtain in this case to aid in the diagnosis and treatment of seizures?

a) Maternal Vitamin A use

b) Maternal Vitamin D use

c) Maternal pyridoxine use

d) Maternal Insulin use

e) Maternal anticoagulant use

Qn. 172

A two year old child's mother is concerned about her "bow legs."

She was breast fed for 6 months and started on solid baby food by 5 months. Now she is eating regular food stuffs; but is a picky eater. On physical examination you find swollen expanded wrists. You are most probably going to order

a) Alkaline phosphatase and calcium levels

b) Acid phosphatase levels

c) Vitamin C levels

d) Hemoglobin electrophoresis

e) Karyotyping

Qn. 173

An infant is placed on Total Parenteral Nutrition with intralipids, aminoacids and hyperosmolar dextrose solution along with vitamins and trace elements.

Which of the following common complication is an effect of such long term parenteral nutrition?

a) Cholestatic jaundice

b) Seizures

c) Autism

d) Adrenoleukodystrophy

e) Cataract

Pediatrics e-MCQ

16. Pediatric Surgery & orthopedics

Qn.174

A three year old child was brought to the clinic after developing pain and inability to move the right elbow. Child was walking along a pedestrian crosswalk when he suddenly threw a tantrum and his father had to drag him to the side of the road before the lights changed to red.

On examination, the child is holding his forearm with the left hand, crying and not allowing anyone to examine him. You do not find any swelling or bruising on the elbow.

Probable diagnosis is

a) Supra condylar fracture of humerus

b) Fracture of olecranon

c) Elbow sprain

d) Subluxated radial head

e) Green stick fracture

Pediatrics e-MCQ

Qn. 175

A fourteen year old boy is complaining about painful swellings over his upper legs appeared after two months into his volleyball practice. The pain was intermittent initially, but now it makes him stop the game and rest. The swelling is getting bigger day by day. On physical examination, you find a tender bony hard prominence below the knee joint, on the upper end of the tibia. No evidence of joint effusion or limitation of movements noted. Your diagnosis is

a) Osteochondroma

b) Ewing's sarcoma

c) Osteogenic sarcoma

d) Bakers cyst

e) Osgood Schlatter's disease

Qn. 176

A teenager was injured while playing football. He was tackled by another player and both fell on each other. He felt excruciating pain in his right knee. He was helped to move out of the field by his team mates. On physical examination, you find the right knee joint is slightly swollen and tender. Flexion and extension is limited because of the pain. The maximum tenderness is on the lateral aspect of the knee joint. Anterior and posterior draw tests negative. No locking of the knee joint was found on rotation and extension.

Your diagnosis is

a) Medial meniscus tear

b) Anterior cruciate ligament tear

c) Posterior cruciate ligament tear

d) Lateral meniscus tear

e) Lateral collateral ligament injury

Qn. 177

A sixteen year old, who was riding an all - terrain vehicle, fell on the ground when the vehicle hit a rock. He is now complaining of pain in the right wrist below the base of thumb. His pain is worse on flexion of the wrist joint. On examination, his right wrist joint is slightly swollen. There is tenderness in the anatomical snuff box area. No tenderness on the thumb or fingers. Movements of the wrist thumb are within normal range. You obtain a radiograph of the wrist and the hand, but did not see any fractures.

Your diagnosis is

a) Dislocated carpo metacarpal joint of the first digit

b) Fracture along the growth plate of the radius

c) Fracture of the scaphoid bone

d) Colles fracture

e) Sprain of the abductor pollicis muscle

Qn. 178

A nine month old is admitted with fever, vomiting and abdominal distension. According to the mother, he had few stools with a tinge of blood in it. The child sometimes cries suddenly, becomes irritable and lethargic. He is refusing feeds. You get an x-ray of abdomen, which showed air fluid levels. Your next step in the management of this child's problem is

Pediatrics e-MCQ

a) A barium enema

b) Stool culture

c) Stool ova and parasite testing

d) Technetium scan

e) Colonoscopy

Qn.179

A three month old infant is brought by parent to your office after being seen in the emergency department two days earlier. He was found to have bright red colored stools for many days. He is on soy based formula and there is no similar illness in the family. Physical examination was unremarkable and no anal fissures or lesions noted. Results of stool culture, ova and parasites were normal. Abdominal x-ray was unremarkable.

Your next plan is to

a) Switch formula to regular formula.

b) Start empirical antibiotic treatment

c) Perform a HIV test

d) Arrange a colonoscopy

e) Arrange a Meckel scan

Qn. 180

A nine year old girl is admitted with fever, vomiting, loose stools, right lower quadrant abdominal pain and severe guarding and tenderness on examination. A clinical diagnosis of acute appendicitis was made and an appendectomy was performed. Post operatively the appendix was found to be normal. Which of the following pathogens produce infections which fits this clinical picture?

a) Campylobacter

b) Yersinia entero colitica

c) Shigella

d) E.Coli

e) Rotavirus

Pediatrics e-MCQ

Qn. 181

Congenital diaphragmatic hernia causes severe respiratory compromise in the affected newborns. The commonest site of hernia is found to be at

a) Left Posterolateral location

b) Right anterolateral location

c) Left anterolateral location

d) Retrosternal location

e) Right Posterolateral location

Qn. 182

A seven year old boy was brought to your clinic for the evaluation of a limp on walking noted two days earlier. On physical examination, he was afebrile. There was limitation of abduction and internal rotation of the left hip with a diffuse tenderness. There was some apparent shortening of the left lower limb with positive Trendelenburg gait. On standing on left side, pelvis drops on the right side.

Your provisional diagnosis is

a) Slipped capital femoral epiphysis

b) Perthes disease

c) Toxic synovitis

d) Septic arthritis of hip

e) Rheumatic fever

Qn.183

A thirteen year old African American boy was brought to the office by his mother when he complained about pain in the right hip for three days. He gives a history of sudden hip pain when he jumped of the school bus one month ago. He does not participate in any sports and denied any history of trauma or sickle cell disease. On examination, you find an obese boy in no apparent discomfort. There is no tenderness on the hip joints. There is limitation of movements of the right hip in all directions because of the pain.

When you flex his hip, the thighs go in lateral rotation.

Your diagnosis is

a) Malingering

b) Slipped femoral capital epiphysis

c) Perthes disease

d) Tuberculosis of hip joint

e) Inter trochanteric fracture of femur

Qn.184

A six week old infant developed profuse vomiting after every feed. He was always hungry and took up to 4 ounces of regular formula every time. After he developed the vomiting episodes, he was fed smaller quantities every two hourly. He was kept in upright position and formula was thickened with rice cereal; but the child did not improve. He was brought to the emergency room where he was found to be mildly jaundiced and dehydrated. In the ER, the child vomited the oral rehydration solution. The vomiting was described as projectile and "like a fountain." CBC showed wbc count of 15,000/cmm with 62% lymphocytes. Hb was 16g/dL and Hct 49%. BMP showed hypokalemia and alkalosis. Total Serum bilirubin was 6mg/dL. An ultra sonogram of the abdomen showed elongated pylorus of 19 mm and thickness of 6 mm.

Your diagnosis is

a) Malrotation

b) Duodenal atresia

c) Hypertrophic pyloric stenosis

d) Intussusception

e) Gastro esophageal reflux

Qn.185

A five year old boy fell from a Monkey bar and hurt his elbow. He was seen in the emergency room after two hours of the incident. The left elbow was swollen and tender to touch and movements were restricted with pain.

A radiograph of the elbow did not reveal any fractures. There was positive fat pad sign and soft tissue swelling.

What would you advice this child?

a) He needs to be seen by an orthopedic specialist for plaster casting and hospitalization for observation

b) He can use an arm sling for two weeks till the swelling is resolved

c) He can be discharged home on a posterior splint and analgesics

d) He does not need any treatment other than ice compress and elevation

e) He needs reduction of subluxated radial head by sudden flexion of the elbow

Pediatrics e-MCQ

Qn.186

An infant was born after normal spontaneous delivery to a mother who had polyhydramnios. Infant established normal respirations soon after the delivery. He was noted to have copious oral secretions in the mouth. Nurse passed an orogastric tube for suctioning, but did not get much secretions. Later on the infant was fed 10 mL of regular formula and suddenly he developed choking and respiratory distress.

What is the probable diagnosis in this infant?

a) Diaphragmatic hernia

b) Tracheo esophageal fistula

c) Pharyngeal diverticulum

d) Gastro esophageal reflux

e) Infant Botulism

Qn.187

A one week old infant is seen in the emergency room with intermittent crying, lethargy and bilious vomiting. Examination of abdomen did not reveal any masses, but there was diffuse tenderness and distension. An erect

Pediatrics e-MCQ

radiograph of abdomen showed dilated stomach and duodenum. Your diagnosis is

a) Hypertrophic pyloric stenosis

b) Gastro esophageal reflux

c) Duodenal atresia

d) Mid gut volvulus

e) Intussusception

Qn.188

A one day old infant with features of Down's syndrome developed bilious vomiting. An ultra sound scan of upper abdomen revealed normal findings. A radiograph of abdomen showed "double bubble" appearance.

Your diagnosis is

a) Pyloric stenosis

b) Malrotation

c) Duodenal atresia

d) Short left colon

e) Hirschsprung disease

Qn.189

An infant had delay in passage of meconium for 40 hours of birth.

Abdominal radiograph showed distended bowel loops. No meconium plug was passed. Barium enema showed a proximal dilated bowel and a narrow distal colon.

Your diagnosis is

a) Cystic fibrosis

b) Short left colon

c) Intussusception

d) Hirschsprung disease

e) Malrotation

Pediatrics e-MCQ

Qn.190

A five year old child was found to be having an absent testis on the left side. His mother said she was not told about this abnormality by any physicians before.

You could not palpate any swelling on the inguinal or pubic areas. You are advising the parent that

a) No investigations because this child is born with one testis only.

b) This will cause a decrease in sperm count when he gets older, but otherwise no problems

c) You will order a nuclear scan of the abdomen to identify the missing testis

d) Identification and orchiopexy is only for cosmetic reasons

e) You will order a CT scan and refer him to urologist for removal of the undescended testis

Qn.191

An infant was born with a cleft lip and palate. Which of the following statements is NOT true regarding this problem?

a) These children are more prone to develop ear infections

b) Cleft lip and palate are surgically corrected at birth simultaneously

c) This shows multifactorial inheritance.

d) Trisomy 18 is associated with cleft lip and palate

e) Infants with these problems should also be screened for associated malformations.

17. Pulmonology

Pediatrics e-MCQ

Qn.192

A 3 month old infant was brought to the clinic with concerns about a noise heard while breathing. The sound occurs in inspiration, mostly while sleeping. He does not have any difficulty in breathing. He was found to be having intermittent bouts of vomiting after feeding since birth.

Your diagnosis is

a) Tracheo esophageal fistula

b) Laryngomalacia

c) Bronchomalacia

d) Pulmonary sequestration

e) Laryngotracheobronchitis

Pediatrics e-MCQ

Qn.193

A 3 year old child is admitted with 3rd episode of pneumonia since birth. The following initial work ups are indicated in finding the etiology of the child's problem, EXCEPT

a) Sweat Chloride test

b) Immunoglobulin levels

c) Antibodies against Tetanus and Diphtheria

d) Complement levels

e) Anti neutrophil cytoplasmic antibodies

Qn. 194

A seven year old is admitted to PICU with status asthmaticus. He is currently on nebulized albuterol and intravenous methyl prednisolone.

The following medications can be useful adjuncts in the management of acute asthma in this child, EXCEPT :

a) Ketamine

b) Halothane

c) Ipratropium bromide

d) Nitric oxide

e) Magnesium sulfate

Qn.195

A child is having cough and wheezing during the Winter months, especially when he goes out in the cold. You suspect hyper reactive airways. Airway hyper reactivity in children can be diagnosed using

a) Methacholine

b) Helium oxygen mixture

c) Antihistamine

d) Atropine

e) Pilocarpine

Pediatrics e-MCQ

Qn.196

A 9 month old is admitted with fever, difficulty breathing and rhinorrhea. She was given nebulized Albuterol every two hours. Her fever resolved after admission, but cough continued. Physical examination revealed inspiratory and expiratory wheezing in both lung fields equally.

CBC showed wbc count of 11,000/cmm with lymphocytic predominance. Her oxygen saturation by pulse oxymetry was 96%. Chest X-ray showed hyperinflation in both lung fields. Six hours after admission, the pulse oxymetry showed oxygen saturation at 88%, without much improvement by O2 given via nasal cannula. Examination of the chest revealed decreased wheezing on the right side compared to the left. Repeat chest X-ray showed opacification of right lung field with slight mediastinal shift to right side.

Your diagnosis is

a) Pneumothorax

b) Mucus plug causing atelectasis

c) Worsening lobar pneumonia

d) Radiological artifact

e) Aspiration pneumonia

Pediatrics e-MCQ

Qn.197

An infant was born with Apgar counts of 8 and 9 at 1 and 5 minutes respectively after a normal spontaneous vaginal delivery. When he was fed a formula by bottle, he suddenly developed respiratory distress. Nurses stopped feeding him and given him O2 via head box; then he regained normal color. He did not have tachypnea, tachycardia or murmurs. SpO2 was 100% in both upper and lower extremities. A radiograph of chest showed normal findings.

Most probable cause of respiratory distress in this new born is

a) Diaphragmatic hernia

b) Tracheoesophageal fistula

c) Choanal atresia

d) Persistent pulmonary hypertension

e) Right to left shunt

18. Rheumatology

Pediatrics e-MCQ

Qn.198

A teenager was seen in the clinic with history of purpuric spots on the body.

She had some rash on the face developed after a soft ball game during the weekend, which she thinks that due to sunburn.

On physical examination, you find wide spread purpuric spots over the ankles and elbows. A scaly erythematous malar rash present. Physical examination otherwise was unremarkable.

CBC showed wbc count 5,000/cmm, Polymorphs 63% Lymphocytes 30% Eosinophils 4%, Hb 10.2 mg/dL, Hct 33, Platelets 75,000/cmm.

Your next plan is to do the following, EXCEPT

a) Bone marrow aspiration biopsy

b) Anti-nuclear antibodies

c) Antibodies to double stranded DNA

d) Factor VIII level

e) PTT

Qn.199

A child was seen in the clinic with painful knee joints for three weeks. There is a history of intermittent fever and malaise since the onset of his illness.

On physical examination, he is afebrile, has few lymph nodes on the cervical area and splenic enlargement of 3 cm from the left costal margin.

CBC showed normocytic anemia and wbc count of 5,000/cmm with poly 55% lymph 40% and monocytes 4% ESR is 24

What is your diagnosis?

a) Acute rheumatic fever

b) SLE

c) Juvenile rheumatoid arthritis

d) Lyme disease

e) Brucellosis

Pediatrics e-MCQ

Qn.200

A ten year old boy is complaining of weakness, especially when he gets up from sitting position, climbing stairs etc. for two weeks. He was taking over the counter analgesics, without much benefit. He recently developed a purple rash over his eye lids. You suspect this as a case of Juvenile Dermatomyositis. Which of the following feature you would find on his nails?

a) Splinter hemorrhages

b) Periungual fibroma

c) Beau's lines

d) Pitting

e) Nail fold telangiectasia

Qn. 201

A seventeen year old girl was diagnosed to have pelvic inflammatory disease and was started on Doxycycline. A week later, she developed an erythematous rash over the face and pain in the small joints of the hand. A provisional diagnosis of SLE was made. Which of the following is a true statement regarding SLE?

a) If anti-nuclear antibodies are present, the diagnosis is confirmed

b) Drug induced SLE is present if Anti-ds DNA and Anti-Sm are positive

c) SLE characteristically shows low Complement (C3, C4) levels

d) SLE is usually associated with low anti phospholipid antibodies

e) Anti-smith antibodies correspond to the activity of SLE

Qn.202

Which of the following is a true statement regarding juvenile rheumatoid arthritis (JRA)?

a) Rheumatoid factor is negative in children compared to adults

b) Atlanto axial subluxation is a usual complication of JRA

c) Keratoderma blenorrhagicum is a skin manifestation characteristic of JRA

d) Children with uveitis are commonly ANA positive

e) In JRA, the disease process involve only the synovium; bones are unaffected

Pediatrics e-MCQ

Critiques and Answers

Pediatrics e-MCQ

1. Cardiology

Qn.1 Answer is: b

Diaphragmatic hernia usually presents with increasing respiratory distress at birth, with scaphoid abdomen and decreased breath sounds unilaterally. A chest X-ray may be helpful in the diagnosis. Hypoplastic left heart syndrome tend to be symptomatic as the ductus arteriosus closes physiologically. This causes a sudden decrease in systemic perfusion as it was dependent on the right heart and features of circulatory failure ensue. Tetralogy of Fallot does not typically follow this course. Necrotizing entero colitis can cause abdominal distension, apneas, feeding intolerance and heme positive stools in usually premature infants and those with hypoxia. Galactosemia does not manifest as circulatory shock.

Qn.2 Answer is b.

This infant has symptomatic supra ventricular tachycardia, which needs to be diagnosed early and should be treated.

Pediatrics e-MCQ

There is respiratory distress which is due to cardiac failure. The treatment involves intravenous Adenosine. Closure of the Ductus Arteriosus usually manifests in children with Ductus dependent lesions like the hypoplastic left heart syndrome and can be delayed for few days. Lupus in the mother can manifest as bradycardia in the infant.

Qn.3 Answer is a.

Persistent pulmonary hypertension can produce worsening of symptoms when the pulmonary resistance is increased as well as venous return is impeded. Post ductal hypoxemia is characteristic. PPHN can also be associated with congenital cardiac as well as lung malformations. Transposition of great arteries presents with hypoxemia, unchanged with 100% FiO2. Pulmonary sequestration usually presents with findings similar to infection and with abnormalities in chest X-ray, as is congenital lobar emphysema. Transient tachypnea of newborn is common in infants born to Diabetic mothers and lasts less than 24 hours.

Qn. 4 Answer is c.

Pediatrics e-MCQ

DiGeorge syndrome is characterized by abnormal facies, hypoplasia or aplasia of parathyroid, thymus and cardiac malformations. Williams's syndrome can have supravalvar aortic stenosis, long philtrum, but hypercalcemia is seen. Noonan syndrome presents with high arched palate, short neck, atrial septal defect or pulmonic stenosis. Hypocalcaemia is not characteristic in Fetal alcohol syndrome and Marfan syndrome, even though there can be craniofacial abnormalities.

Qn.5. Answer is b.

Myocarditis in children follows mostly entero viral infections like Coxsackie virus. Acute onset circulatory shock and respiratory distress is commonly seen

Qn. 6 Answer is d.

The most common association with Lithium use in pregnancy is Ebstein's anomaly, a prolapse of the tricuspid valve into the right ventricle. Coarctation of aorta, patent ductus arteriosus , endocardial cushion defect and congenital heart block are not linked to Lithium use during pregnancy.

Pediatrics e-MCQ

Qn.7 Answer is c.

Heart block in newborns is associated with maternal history of SLE

Qn.8 Answer is d.

Reversible septal hypertrophy often seen in large for gestational age infants was born to a mother with gestational diabetes. There other congenital heart defects like ventricular septal defect and transposition are also seen, but to a lesser degree.

Qn.9 Answer is C.

A soft blowing systolic ejection murmur of intensity grade II/VI at the left sternal border which changes intensity with posture is consistent with functional murmur and is of no clinical significance

Pediatrics e-MCQ

Qn.10 Answer is a.

A systolic murmur at the apex with a mid-systolic click is associated with mitral valve prolapse. As per the latest recommendations of American Heart Association, patients with asymptomatic mitral valve prolapse do not need any endocarditis prophylaxis

Qn. 11 Answer is C.

A decompensation occurring after viral upper respiratory tract infection and cardiac shadow appearing like 'Snow Man" or "figure of 8" is very much suggestive of total anomalous pulmonary venous return. Tetralogy of Fallot typically have "Boot shaped heart" in chest x-rays.

Ebstein's anomaly will show right atrial hypertrophy pattern.

Transposition shows cardiac shadow as "egg on a string" appearance with narrow mediastinum. Pulmonary embolism does not have any specific findings in routine radiographs.

Qn. 12 Answer is d.

Endocardial cushion defect or atrio ventricular canal defect is the commonest cardiac abnormality seen in patients with Down's syndrome.

Turner's syndrome is associated with coarctation. Williams syndrome is associated with supra valvar aortic stenosis

Qn. 13 Answer is C.

A right ventricular hypertrophy pattern with right ventricular conduction delay and right axis deviation is characteristic of atrial septal defect of the secundum type. In ASD primum type, a left axis deviation is seen.

Qn.14 Answer is e.

Tetralogy of Fallot consists of the following four anomalies of the heart :

Right ventricular hypertrophy, Overriding dextropositioned aorta, Infundibular pulmonary stenosis and ventricular septal defect.

Pediatrics e-MCQ

Shunting through patent ductus arteriosus is not seen.

Qn. 15 Answer is e.

Cyanosis is not the presenting feature of Coarctation of Aorta as there is no right to left shunting.

Pediatrics e-MCQ

2. Child Psychiatry

Qn. 16 Answer is e.

Clonidine, an alpha agonist is used in the treatment of ADHD and tics. The side effect of sedation is therapeutically beneficial in children with ADHD having sleep problems.

Qn.17 Answer is a.

Aggravation of tics is commonly seen as a side effect of stimulant therapy. Children usually show poor weight gain. There is no added increase in seizures with concomitant Albuterol treatment or aggravation of asthma. Cardiac arrhythmias are not significantly seen more than general population, even though caution should be exercised in patients with pre-existing heart disease

Pediatrics e-MCQ

Qn.18 Answer is d.

Commonly known drug of abuse, 'Ecstasy' is an amphetamine, chemically MDMA (3,4-methylenedioxy-N-methylamphetamine)

Poisoning with amphetamines is common in adolescents.

The features of overdose are that of adrenergic over activity.

Qn.19 Answer is d.

Many inventories and questionnaires are used in clinical practice to assess the ADHD symptoms and to rule out comorbid conditions like depression, anxiety, learning disabilities, oppositional defiant disorder and conduct disorder. The features described in the vignette are pointing towards oppositional defiant disorder and conduct disorder of childhood onset.

Qn. 20 Answer is b.

Lithium can cause hypothyroidism and thyroid function tests should be done periodically while on the treatment. Goiter is commonly seen in people treated with Lithium. Inhibition of coupling of iodotyrosine residues to form iodothyronines (T3 and T4) and inhibition of release of T4 and T3 are thought to be responsible for the anti-thyroid effects.

Qn.21 Answer is d.

Anorexia nervosa is characterized by multi organ dysfunction and features like high cortisol, pancreatitis, superior mesenteric artery syndrome, cardiac failure and hypocalcaemia.

Qn.22 Answer is a.

Autistic spectrum disorder is characterized by significant deficits in cognitive, social, language and adaptive functioning domains as well as show presence of rigid behaviors, preoccupation with restricted range of interests, lack of spontaneous imaginary play, ritualistic activity and stereotypies.

There is high incidence of seizures, which is not however a clinical diagnostic criterion.

Pediatrics e-MCQ

3. Emergency Medicine

Qn.23 Answer is c.

Iron is toxic in high quantities. A 20-30 mg/Kg dose can cause gastrointestinal effects like vomiting, diarrhea and abdominal pain. 40-60 mg/Kg dose can result in shock and coma and doses over 60 mg/Kg are lethal to children. A serum iron level should be obtained at 4 hours of ingestion. It is useful to visualize iron pill fragments before and after gastric lavage. Desferoxamine is indicated in symptomatic patients or serum levels are more than 500 microgram/dL. Hemodialysis is indicated in renal failure to remove the iron-chelator complex.

Qn. 24 Answer is b.

An unconscious victim found in this scenario should be suspected of having a cervical trauma also unless proved otherwise. Seizures could also result in injury. A normally breathing patient should be just provided supportive care. Simple eyelid myokymia or focal seizures should not be aggressively treated unless you are suspecting status epilepticus. Giving gastric lavage may be dangerous in individuals with coma and defective gag reflux.

Qn.25 Answer is b.

She needs to have her Acetaminophen levels checked every 4 hours. N Acetyl cysteine is administered every 4 hours until the levels are nontoxic.

Qn. 26 Answer is b.

Button cell batteries are liable to corrosion and breakage in the stomach and intestinal tract, potentially releasing toxic chemicals unlike the ingested coins. It can also cause severe burns of the esophagus. In case of ingestion of very small batteries without any magnet co-ingestion in children older than 12 years, asymptomatic cases may be observed at home by vigilant parents. For specific algorithm, please consult national poison center.

Pediatrics e-MCQ

Qn. 27 Answer is c.

This scenario is highly typical for a congenital heart disease which is ductus arteriosus dependent for systemic perfusion (e.g. Hypoplastic left heart syndrome). As the ductus is closing, the infant is facing circulatory shock. The prostaglandin infusion can prevent the closure of ductus and can divert the blood to aorta and can stabilize the patient till infant gets definitive surgery. Rest of the options is not indicated.

Qn.28 Answer is a.

Nonspecific symptoms and signs in a child of this age are suspicious for abuse. Mongolian spots are very common over lumbar and buttock regions in children who are pigmented by racial origin. A retinal hemorrhage however, in this age group is pathognomonic of abusive head trauma. While ruling out other possibilities, physical abuse should be considered first and order appropriate imaging studies.

Qn. 29 Answer is c.

Pediatrics e-MCQ

Many of the children who are exclusively fed on diluted formula are liable to develop hyponatremia.

This has been observed in inner city children who are cared by mothers from poor socioeconomic situations. Mothers who are drug users sell the WIC provided infant formula to the black market for purchasing drugs of abuse. The children are then fed more diluted formulae resulting in symptomatic hyponatremia.

Qn.30 Answer is d.

Carbon monoxide poisoning is very common in households with faulty ventilation from heaters. Sometimes people who are using gas/coal/wood burning fire places do not recognize that the carbon monoxide levels are dangerously high and that can be lethal.

Initial symptoms of low carbon monoxide poisoning could be non-specific symptoms like headache, malaise and lethargy.

Pulse oxymeter will show normal oxygen saturation. Having a high degree of suspicion for potential toxicities like carbon monoxide poisoning is very important in clinical practice.

Pediatrics e-MCQ

Qn. 31 Answer is e.

In submersion victims, the commonest electrocardiographic rhythm seen is asystole.

Pediatrics e-MCQ

4. Endocrinology

Qn. 32 Answer is d.

Congenital adrenal hyperplasia is routinely screened during the newborn screening panel adopted by many states these days. Increased sex steroids can present with virilization, as this female infant showings increase in the androgenic effect.

Qn.33 Answer is c

This girl showing delayed puberty without onset of menstruation or gonadal development should be screened for genetic conditions like Turners syndrome.

Qn. 34 Answer is b.

Hashimoto's thyroiditis or chronic lymphocytic thyroiditis is common auto immune thyroiditis. This causes goiter with hypothyroid and intermittent hyperthyroid states. This is the commonest cause of hypothyroidism in USA.

Pediatrics e-MCQ

Qn. 35 Answer is a.

Nuclear disasters release radioactive Iodine isotopes into the environment, which will eventually get trapped in the thyroid gland, exposing the person to malignant transformation in the gland. Papillary carcinoma of thyroid is commonly seen.

Qn. 36 Answer is c.

To replace the losses due to osmotic diuresis and to avoid acidosis due to excess chloride.

Qn.37 Answer is c.

Acanthosis nigricans is the pigmentation seen over neck and axilla. This is commonly seen in people with hyper insulinism and insulin resistance. It is also seen in obesity and can also be familial trait.

Pediatrics e-MCQ

Qn.38 Answer is c.

For the treatment for refractory hypoglycemia, Diazoxide is used

Qn. 39 Answer is e.

Exogenous Insulin administration can be a cause of hypoglycemia, which was noted in conditions of Munchausen syndrome by proxy and C-Peptide levels will be low, unless in Insulinoma, there will be elevated Insulin and C-peptide levels.

Qn.40 Answer is a.

Irregular menstruation, obesity, hirsutism, acne are features of poly cystic ovary syndrome

Pediatrics e-MCQ

Qn.41 Answer is d.

Auto immune poly glandular disease is characterized by hypoparathyroidism, mucocutaneous candidiasis, pernicious anemia and Addison disease. However, Pheochromocytoma is not seen(but it may be part of multiple endocrine neoplasia syndrome/MEN)

Qn.42 Answer is d.

SIADH can follow head trauma. This will be manifested by hyponatremia and low osmolality. Fluid restriction is indicated to bring serum sodium over 130 mEq/L

5. Gastroenterology

Qn.43 Answer is c.

Lactase deficiency is manifested as bloating, diarrhea and intolerance to feeds. Stools are positive for reducing substances and can be acidic. This causes excoriation in the perianal region.

Qn.44 Answer is e.

An elevated conjugated hyperbilirubinemia characterized by increased direct bilirubin at this age is suggestive of liver disease. Among all the listed options, Alpha 1 antitrypsin deficiency is the condition which causes direct hyperbilirubinemia. Other options listed are causes of unconjugated hyperbilirubinemia

Pediatrics e-MCQ

Qn. 45 Answer is d

Lactose intolerance can be primary or secondary. Galactosemia is not associated with lactose intolerance. Stool pH in lactose intolerance is acidic due to conversion of lactose to lactic acid. Lactose intolerance can occur after an infection with Giardia and also viral gastro enteritis .Dermatitis Herpetiformes is the skin condition associated with Gluten sensitivity, not with lactose intolerance.

Qn.46 Answer is C.

Anti-tissue transglutaminase antibodies or anti-endomyseum antibodies are considered to be most specific for Celiac disease.

Qn.47 Answer is b.

High serum gastrin levels , gastric hyper secretion and peptic ulcerations are seen in Systemic Mastocytosis. This condition is due to proliferation of mastocytes in extra cutaneous tissues like bone marrow, gastro intestinal tract including stomach, liver and spleen.

Pediatrics e-MCQ

Qn. 48 Answer is c.

Excessive fruit juice consumption could be a cause of protracted diarrhea and malabsorption. Parents should be queried specifically for this history in any child with diarrhea

Qn.49 Answer is c.

Anorexia nervosa should be a diagnosis kept in mind when there is significant weight loss in a teenager. Most of the cases, the weight loss, diarrhea and vomiting are not however, brought up as presenting complaints. Crohn's disease is one of the commonest cause for this typical presentation.

Qn.50 Answer is d.

A stool immune assay for Giardia is the most sensitive test for diagnosis of Giardia lamblia infection.

Qn.51 Answer is b.

Pediatrics e-MCQ

Urease in the stomach used to split urea by Helicobacter pylori can be assessed by using non-radioactive C13 labeled urea. This test is noninvasive.

Qn.52 Answer is b.

Esophageal pH probe is a widely used sensitive test to diagnose gastro esophageal reflux in this age group.

Qn.53 Answer is C

Untreated chronic constipation with fecal impaction in the rectum can manifest as intermittent watery stools and fecal soiling. Increasing fiber in diet is not going to resolve this unless a good bowel clean out is done using laxatives.

Qn.54 Answer is e.

Steroids and other immunosuppressive treatments are used in the treatment of Crohn's disease.

Pediatrics e-MCQ

Qn.55 Answer is d.

An unconjugated hyperbilirubinemia which is manifested during stress and fasting states is commonly seen in patients with Gilbert's Syndrome. They are mostly asymptomatic individuals and levels of bilirubin are not usually high and have no other evidence of hepatic dysfunction. No treatment is necessary.

Qn.56 Answer is c.

Ileal resections or short bowel syndrome can cause various deficiency states and malabsorption. Vitamin B12 deficiency is a consequence of terminal ileal resection.

Qn.57 Answer is b.

There are many causes for protein losing enteropathy. Stool alpha 1 antitrypsin spot test is a non-invasive test widely used to diagnose this condition. D-xylose absorption test and Breath hydrogen test are tests for malabsorption of sugars.

Qn.58 Answer is a.

Cow's milk protein allergy can present with bloody diarrhea, rash and wheezing.

Pediatrics e-MCQ

Rest of the options listed do not have this clinical spectrum

6. Genetics

Qn. 59 Answer is d.

Turner syndrome is manifested in girls as growth failure, webbed neck, gonadal failure, cardiac abnormalities like coarctation of aorta and bicuspid aortic valve and high incidence of renal abnormalities, especially horse shoe kidney. Karyotyping reveals one X chromosome being absent.

Qn.60 Answer is d.

Fetal alcohol syndrome is characterized by widely spaced eyes, thin lips.

Fetal hydantoin syndrome is characterized by microcephaly, abnormalities of digits and nails. Edwards syndrome is trisomy 18, associated with cleft lip and palate, umbilical hernia, cardiac abnormalities and rocker bottom feet.

Pediatrics e-MCQ

Qn.61 Answer is b.

Individuals with Prader-Willi syndrome commonly have failure to thrive in early infancy, which will later change to voracious appetite and leading to obesity. They also have hypotonia and rudimentary genitalia. Genes in chromosome 15 are deleted and this condition is associated with imprinting.

Qn.62 Answer is b.

Angelman syndrome is an example of genomic imprinting, that is caused by deletion or inactivation of genes on the maternally inherited chromosome 15 while the paternal copy, which may be of normal sequence, is imprinted and therefore silenced. Affected individuals have developmental delay, "happy puppet-like" demeanor and gait.

Qn.63 Answer is c.

Uniparental disomy is present when both chromosomes of a pair of chromosomes are inherited from a single parent.

Pediatrics e-MCQ

Genomic imprinting is seen when the phenotypic expression of the offspring depends on which parent the chromosome or genes originated. Classical example of imprinting is Angelman syndrome and Pradder-Willi syndrome

Qn.64 Answer is b.

Lesch-Nyhan syndrome is a X-linked disorder of purine metabolism due to the absence or deficiency of hypoxanthine guanine phospho ribosyl transferase, and is characterized by self-mutilation, developmental delays, dystonic movements and propensity to have uric acid stones in the kidneys

Qn. 65 Answer is b.

Patients with Marfan syndrome have tall body habitus, pectus excavatum, heart valve abnormalities and have risk of developing spontaneous pneumothorax

Qn.66 Answer is a.

Pediatrics e-MCQ

William's syndrome is characterized by hypercalcaemia in early infancy, facial dysmorphism and supra valvar aortic stenosis. They are at risk for developmental delays. They seem to have a very outgoing personality.

Qn. 67 Answer is b.

Fragile X syndrome is a triple nucleotide repeat disorder, which is a common cause of mental retardation after Down's syndrome. There are certain physical features like large ears, tall stature and macro orchidism associated with this condition.

Qn.68 Answer is b.

Kallmann Syndrome is associated with tall stature and anosmia

Qn. 69 Answer is a.

Trisomy 18, Edwards syndrome is associated with microcephaly, short sternum, micrognathia, narrow hips and a rocker-bottom feet.

Qn.70 Answer is b.

An inferiorly dislocated lens (in Marfan it is superiorly dislocated), tall stature, scoliosis, pectus excavatum and pes planus are seen in Homocystinuria. It can share some features of mar fan's syndrome

Qn. 71 Answer is c.

Achondroplasia is associated with short stature and abnormal limbs. Fractures are not characteristic. Child has osteogenesis imperfecta

Rickets and Vitamin C deficiency do not produce recurrent fractures, even though skeletal growth abnormalities are seen.

Pediatrics e-MCQ

Qn. 72 Answer is a.

Fluorescent in-situ Hybridization (FISH)test is used to diagnose suspected for DiGeorge Syndrome (FISH 22q11-). DiGeorge anomaly/velocardiofacial syndrome (DG/VCFS) occurs with different deletion intervals on chromosomes 22q11, while the DiGeorge anomaly (with other findings) is seen in patients with deletions of 10p14.

Qn.73 Answer is b.

Beckwith-Weidemann syndrome is associated with Tumors, including Wilm's Tumor. There are other findings like macroglossia, microcephaly and earlobe fissures. Beckwith-Weidemann syndrome is associated with Tumors, including Wilm's Tumor

Pediatrics e-MCQ

7. Growth and Development

Qn. 74 Answer is d.

A four year old is not expected to tandem walk.

Qn.75 Answer is a.

Moro reflex and Asymmetric tonic neck reflex are seen in the young infants and are classified as primitive reflexes. However persistence beyond certain age, asymmetry or incomplete Moro reflex are considered abnormal and can give clues to neuro developmental abnormalities.

Qn.76 Answer is b.

A four year old is able to copy a circle and a square, but not a triangle

Pediatrics e-MCQ

Qn.77 Answer is c.

At 3 years, children are able to stack blocks to make bridge shape.

Qn.78 Answer is c.

A female child with microcephaly, developmental delay, anxiety, hyperventilation and loss of acquired purposeful hand movements is suggestive of Rett's syndrome. They have characteristic handwringing movements and significant language delay

Pediatrics e-MCQ

8. Hematology and Oncology

Qn.79 Answer is c.

Patients on anticoagulation should be watched for sudden neurological deficits and signs of bleeding. Anticoagulant induced hematoma compressing the nerve trunks is the reason in this case.

Qn.80 Answer is a.

vonWillebrand disease is one of the commonest bleeding disorders manifested in childhood. History of excessive bleeding after surgery, epistaxis etc. are seen. Qualitative and quantitative deficiency of the vonWillebrand factor is responsible.

Qn.81 Answer is b.

Immune thrombocytopenic purpura can follow viral infections. There is reduction in the platelet count, which at times can be refractory. Absence of anemia and abnormal white blood cell count rules out bone marrow infiltration and leukemia. Henoch Schonlein purpura shows normal and elevated platelet counts, symptoms like arthralgia, abdominal pain, intestinal hemorrhage.

Qn.82 Answer is a.

Febrile neutropenic patients who had chemotherapy should be admitted to hospital for broad spectrum antibiotic treatment as sepsis can be overwhelming and life threatening in these patients.

Qn.83 Answer is c.

Splenic sequestration crisis can be seen in patients with sickle cell disease. There is significant splenomegaly with low platelet counts are seen.

Pediatrics e-MCQ

Qn. 84 Answer is e.

Sickle Thalassemia can be manifested as chronic anemia. Hemoglobin electrophoresis will help to diagnose this condition

Qn.85 Answer is a.

Lymphomas manifest as enlarged lymph nodes in the cervical and axillary region. There can also be mediastinal lymphadenopathy detected in the chest radiographs.

Qn.86 Answer is a.

G6PD deficiency is manifested as neonatal hyperbilirubinemia. Hemolysis is seen in the affected individuals when exposed to certain drugs and chemicals. G6 PD deficiency is prevalent in certain ethnic populations. Other options listed are also causes of hyperbilirubinemia.

Qn.87 Answer is b.

Pediatrics e-MCQ

Tumor lysis syndrome is commonly seen in cancer patients. This is characterized by elevated uric acid and potassium levels. IV hydration, alkalinization and Allopurinol are mainstays of management.

Qn.88 answer is a.

Acute Intermittent porphyria is an autosomal dominant disorder affecting the production of heme, the oxygen-binding prosthetic group of hemoglobin. It is characterized by a deficiency of the enzyme porphobilinogen deaminase. Urinary porphobilinogen levels are the first starting point of testing for porphyria.

Qn.89 Answer is a.

Wilm's tumor can be found in asymptomatic children insidiously due to their size. Neuroblastoma and Phaeochromocytoma are mostly small and may be associated with increased urine catecholamine metabolites. They tend to develop near the sympathetic chain.

Pediatrics e-MCQ

Qn.90 Answer is c.

Langerhans Cell Histiocytosis can mimic different disorders. Some of them are locally invasive. Typical histological picture is useful to distinguish it from lymphomas and leukemias

Qn.91 Answer is d.

Ewing's Sarcoma group of cancers have predilection to ribs and long bones. The characteristic onion skinning pattern of bone destruction and soft tissue swelling is diagnostic.

Pediatrics e-MCQ

9. Immunology & Allergy

Qn. 92 Answer is C

In this vignette the history is typical of allergic rhinitis, particularly the allergic shiners around the eye and bilateral middle ear effusion, a common accompaniment of the ongoing respiratory allergic insults. The onset of cough and superadded purulent nasal discharge makes this more likely to be an acute sinusitis. Chronic nasal congestion leads to mouth breathing and thereby make the tonsils enlarge chronically. A viral upper respiratory infection can produce middle ear effusion, cough and nasal discharge; but the prolonged course, the polymorpho nuclear leukocytosis make that an unlikely diagnosis here.

Retained nasal foreign bodies produce thick purulent, foul smelling nasal discharge in children, but it is usually unilateral unless you have foreign bodies in both nostrils.

Kartagener's syndrome is otherwise called immotile cilia syndrome. It is characterized by recurrent sinusitis, respiratory infections like bronchiectasis and congenital abnormalities like dextrocardia and or situs inversus. We do not have any history here suggesting this rare syndrome; but it is worthwhile considering in the cases of recurrent sino

Pediatrics e-MCQ

pulmonary diseases. IgA deficiency is the commonest type of immunodeficiency in children, incidence about 1/400 children. IgA is the antibody present on the epithelial surfaces and it plays a role in the humoral immunity against gastro intestinal and respiratory infections. Selective IgA deficiency runs as an autosomal dominant trait with variable expression. It is an unlikely diagnosis in this child; but if recurrent respiratory infections occur, An Immunoglobin level should be determined.

Qn.93 Answer is C

In cases of selective IgA deficiency, most of the time you find an elevated IgM level also. These children are prone to gastro intestinal infections and respiratory infections.

There is no history suggestive of T cell dysfunction here. Hence severe combined immuno deficiency is not a likely answer. Since levels of other immunoglobulins are normal, Bruton's agammaglobulinemia is unlikely. X-Linked immunodeficiency with Hyper IgM will have low or normal IgA and low IgG. They most of the time present with respiratory infections. In IgG subclass deficiency, one will not come across elevated IgM and low IgA.

Qn.94 Answer is A

DiGeorge syndrome is characterized by thymic aplasia or hypoplasia. This condition occurs in both males and females. Microdeletions of chromosome 22 (22q11.2) cause multiple abnormalities. Affected children are susceptible to infections due to viruses, fungi and opportunistic pathogens like pneumocystis carinii. T cell function is deficient and most of the time immunoglobulin levels are normal. Thymic transplants and HLA-compatible bone marrow transplantation helps to restore the immunologic function. Since T-cell function cannot be restored by immunoglobulins, that option is wrong. At this time prenatal treatments are not available. Growth hormone treatment or splenectomy cannot bring any change in the immune function.

Qn.95 Answer is D

This child has multiple episodes of deep seated infections due to pyogenic organisms, a history typical of the chronic granulomatous disease(CGD). The disease is due to the defect in intra cellular killing inside the phagocytes. Sweat chloride level is normal in CGD.

Antibody levels to Tetanus and diphtheria denotes a normal T cell function. Absence of thrombocytopenia rules out Wiskott Aldrich Syndrome, which is characterized by thrombocytopenic purpura, atopic dermatitis, and immunodeficiency. They are prone to infections like otitis media due to Pneumococci and other bacteria with polysaccharide capsules. Immunoglobulin levels will be abnormal.

Cystic Fibrosis(CF) is characterized by an abnormality in the chloride transporter gene(CFTR : cystic fibrosis trans membrane regulator). Affected children develop sino pulmonary infections due to the thick viscid secretions. Sweat chloride test with values more than 60 mEq/L is suspicious of Cystic Fibrosis. Pilocarpine iontophoresis is used to produce sweat by passing an electric current through the skin. Adequate amount (at least 50mg) of sweat production is needed to establish the diagnosis. Conditions which can interfere with sweat production will produce false positive results. Infections in CF are mostly due to S. aureus and Pseudomonas.

Complement system is important in the body defense against pathogens like Neisseria. Total hemolytic complement activity(CH50) is a useful screening test of deficiencies.

Asplenia or splenectomy can cause opsonization defects and thereby make the individual susceptible to infections by encapsulated bacteria like pneumococcus.

Pediatrics e-MCQ

Qn.96 Answer is B

Nitro blue tetrazolium test is the diagnostic screening test for chronic granulomatous disease. Dihydroiodine rhodamine flow cytometry tests are employed more recently.

Adenosine deaminase deficiency is a type of severe combined immune deficiency with near normal B cell function and defective T cell function. `They have marked lymphopenia, vertebral and rib cage anomalies. Lymph node biopsy usually employed to diagnose T cell defects.

Qn. 97 Answer is B

Typical history of chronic skin ulcers, delayed umbilical stump dehiscence is characteristic of Leukocyte Adhesion Deficiency(LAD). Leukocyte function in phagocytosis is affected by the inability of neutrophils to migrate to sites of inflammation and intra cellular adhesion. Neutrophil count and delayed immune responses are normal. Treatment is allogenic bone marrow transplant and prophylactic antibiotics.

Pediatrics e-MCQ

Maternal cocaine use is not found to have any relationship with delayed wound healing or umbilical stump dehiscence.

Group B Streptococci (GBS)can produce infections in some newborns, mostly invasive. But majority of colonized infants are asymptomatic.

Child abuse is suspected when there are unexplained burns or patterned wounds in any child. An unbiased history taking and examination in detail will give more insights into the diagnosis than sophisticated tests. But that should not prevent a smart clinician to order tests and investigate further as needed.

Qn.98 Answer C

Flow cytometry for CD11/CD18 surface glycoprotein levels can identify Leukocyte Adhesion Deficiency. The test employs monoclonal antibodies directed against CD11b glycoprotein on Neutrophils

Pediatrics e-MCQ

Qn.99 Answer is D

Ataxia telangiectasia is characterized by the ocular, skin capillary telangiectasia, cerebellar ataxia, Sino pulmonary infections with defect in cellular and humoral immunity. The affected individuals are prone to develop lympho reticular malignancies. They are radio sensitive and are advised to avoid radiation exposure as much as possible. Telangiectasia can develop later in life and other symptoms like ataxia can occur early in childhood.

Myeloperoxidase deficiency is a defect in phagocytes, causing recurrent Candida infections especially seen in Diabetes, but affected individuals can be asymptomatic. Severe combined immuno deficiency is not associated with ataxia or telangiectasia.

Shwachman-Diamond syndrome is an autosomal recessive inherited condition associated with leukopenia, malabsorption, diarrhea, growth failure, dwarfism and delayed puberty. They develop infections due to neutropenia. No association with telangiectasia or ataxia is seen.

Pediatrics e-MCQ

Qn.100 Answer is B

Post nasal drip is a common problem with Allergic Rhinitis. Night time cough can be a symptom of childhood asthma, which is also possible in a child with allergies.

This child is probably allergic to indoor allergens or outdoor allergens. An allergy skin test is the best way to identify the offending allergens. RAST testing is not commonly used these days because it only identifies the IgE against allergens. People with circulating IgE against a particular allergen are sometimes surprisingly asymptomatic on exposure. Skin testing will help to arrange immunotherapy and desensitization, which might be the next step in this child who is already on nasal corticosteroids and antihistamines.

Humidifiers are useless in allergic rhinitis and they cause mold growth and can cause more problems than any actual benefit.

Polysomnogram is used to identify people with sleep apnea and will not benefit this child to control his allergies. This will be useful later to evaluate the possibility of obstructive sleep apnea due to enlarged tonsils, a usual accompaniment of chronic allergic rhinitis and mouth breathing.

10. Infectious Diseases

Qn. 101 Answer is a.

The child described in this scenario has features of Kawasaki syndrome, am immune mediated vasculitis affecting arteries. There is high risk for development of coronary aneurysms and an echocardiogram may be ordered. These children are also prescribed Aspirin.

Qn. 102 Answer is a.

The clinical manifestations in this child are consistent with scarlet fever, due to streptococcus pyogenes infection. There is no evidence of vesicular rash in the mucosa suggestive of herpangina and no erythema migrans of Lyme disease.

Qn. 103 Answer is b.

Pediatrics e-MCQ

Listeria causes meningitis in newborns, a common pathogen mothers get infected usually from contaminated food products like blue cheese. It is treated with Ampicillin. Other causes of meningitis in newborns are Group B streptococcus and E Coli.

Pneumocystis carinii, Cryptococcus neoformans are common etiologies of meningitis in immunocompromized individuals. Candida can cause intra cranial infection in premature newborns on multiple broad spectrum antibiotics.

Qn. 104 Answer is e.

Pseudomonas is not usually associated with acute otitis media. It may be seen in chronic otitis as well as external otitis

Qn. 105 Answer is b.

Palivizumab is a monoclonal antibody that reduces hospitalizations due to RSV infection among children at high-risk for severe disease. It is given in monthly intramuscular injections during the RSV season, which generally lasts from

November through March in most locations in the United States.

According to the AAP, palivizumab prophylaxis may be considered for the following groups of infants and children:

Infants born at 28 weeks' gestation or earlier during RSV season, whenever that occurs during the first 12 months of life

Infants born at 29–32 weeks' gestation if they are younger than 6 months of age at the start of the RSV season

Infants born at 32–35 weeks' gestation who are younger than 3 months of age at the start of the RSV season or who are born during RSV season if they have at least one of the following 2 risk factors: 1) infant attends child care; 2) infant has a sibling younger than 5 years of age

Infants and children younger than 2 years with cyanotic or complicated congenital heart disease

Infants and children younger than 2 years who have been treated for chronic lung disease within 6 months of the start of the RSV season.

Infants born before 35 weeks of gestation who have either congenital abnormalities of the airway or neuromuscular disease that compromises handling of respiratory secretions

Pediatrics e-MCQ

Qn. 106 Answer is d.

Oseltamivir, Zanamivir, Amantadine, Rimantadine are used in the treatment of Influenza. Indinavir is an anti-retroviral medication, a protease inhibitor used in the treatment of HIV infection.

Qn.107 Answer is b.

Lyme disease is very common in many states, not only Wisconsin. The appearance of circular rash Erythema migrans may be initial characteristic feature. However in many individuals, this may get overlooked as the rash does not cause any itching and many do not recall any tick bite.

Qn. 108 Answer is e.

Coxsackie A virus causes fever, mucus membrane vesicles, ulcers and lymphadenopathy. There can also be vesicles on the palmar and plantar surfaces.

Qn.109 Answer is c.

There is an increase in Rabies exposure during expeditions as mentioned in the vignette. Rabid bats have been documented in all 49 continental states. Bats are increasingly implicated as important wildlife reservoirs for variants of rabies virus transmitted to humans. Recent data suggest that transmission of rabies virus can occur from minor, seemingly unimportant, or unrecognized bites from bats. Rabies post-exposure prophylaxis is recommended for all persons with bite, scratch, or mucous membrane exposure to a bat, unless the bat is available for testing and is negative for evidence of rabies.

Qn.110 Answer is a.

Viral load is the definitive test to assess the HIV disease activity in this child.

Qn.111 Answer is a.

Cat scratch fever caused by Bartonella henselae is associated with lymphangitis, lymphadenopathy, headache and fever.

Qn. 112 Answer is d.

This is a classical presentation of tinea capitis, a dermatophytosis, a superficial fungal infection, which is resistant to common topical antifungal agents. As the fungus is growing deep in the hair follicle, it does not get irradicated quickly. Griseofulvin, a systemic antifungal agent is useful.

Qn.113 Answer is c.

Cat bites have increased tendency to get infected. Many species of pathogens present in the oral cavity (e.g. pasteurella) are sensitive to Amoxicillin Clavulanate

Qn. 114 Answer is e.

Bacterial meningitis characterized by neck stiffness, headache, malaise and vomiting can be life threatening if not diagnosed early and treatment initiated.

Qn. 115 Answer is c.

Campylobacter is sensitive to Erythromycin.

Pediatrics e-MCQ

Qn. 116 Answer is b.

Severe allergy to egg, prior history of Guillain Barre syndrome, or anaphylaxis after vaccines like MMR are considered as contra indications. There is a slight risk for worsening of multiple sclerosis after infections. It is, however a relative contraindication and most neurologists recommend administration of influenza vaccine to patients with multiple sclerosis.

Qn.117 Answer is d

Qn. 118 Answer is d.

External otitis (Swimmers' ear) is mostly caused by Pseudomonas

Qn. 119 Answer is a.

Staphylococcus aureus is the commonest pathogen in the causation of osteomyelitis in all children. Salmonella osteomyelitis is the second common cause of osteomyelitis in children with sickle cell disease.

Qn. 120 Answer is c.

Pediatrics e-MCQ

Pneumococcal peritonitis is a known complication in patients with nephrotic syndrome. Renal vein thrombosis can occur in children with nephrotic syndrome, but the manifestation is different.

Qn. 121 Answer is b.

Malaria is common in countries of the Asian subcontinent. Intermittent fever with sweating with splenomegaly can be malaria, which can be diagnosed with the blood smear.

Qn. 122 Answer is b.

Leprosy (Hansen's Disease) is caused by mycobacterium leprae, which is spread mostly by contact with nasal secretions.

Qn. 123 Answer is a.

The incidence of waterborne diseases like Hepatitis A and Typhoid is high in Far East. As these are not common in the USA, immunizations for these disorders are not included in the routine vaccinations. So the child should get Hepatitis A and Typhoid vaccination

Pediatrics e-MCQ

11. Metabolic Disorders

Qn.124 Answer is b.

Galactosemia is associated with hypoglycemia and reducing substances in urine.

There is no evidence of hyperammonemia and lactic acidosis

Qn. 125 Answer is c.

Urea cycle disorders usually do not have acidosis and hyper ammonemia may be seen.

Qn.126 Answer is e.

Low urinary ketones are seen in Medium chain acyl coA dehydrogenase deficiency- MCAD (Fatty acid oxidation disorder)

Pediatrics e-MCQ

Qn. 127 Answer is b.

Homocystinuria is associated with dislocation of the lens, developmental delay, Cataract and also convulsions

Qn. 128 Answer is C

Lesch Nyhan syndrome is due to deficiency of HGPRT enzyme in the purine metabolism, which causes accumulation of uric acid in blood and the kidneys. However the chemical substance thought to cause the neurological damage in these children is Hypoxanthine.

Pediatrics e-MCQ

12. Neonatology

Qn. 129 Answer is a.

1 in 4000 term newborns develop ischemic stroke. This is usually manifested as focal seizures developing in 48 hours of life. This may not be identified unless a MRI imaging is obtained. Physical examination is usually unremarkable

Qn. 130 Answer is c.

Alpha feto protein levels are low in Downs syndrome. It can be elevated in neural tube defects including spina bifida.

Qn. 131 Answer is e.

Delayed cord clamping can cause polycythemia, however prolonged hemorrhage from ruptured umbilical vessels can lead to anemia and shock. Sepsis, jaundice and hypothermia are seen in these infants.

Pediatrics e-MCQ

Qn. 132 Answer is b.

Amniotic fluid volume is dependent on the urine production while in utero and also the ingestion by the infant.

Qn. 133 Answer is a.

Necrotizing enterocolitis has multifactorial etiology. This includes prematurity, hypoxia, sepsis and early feeding. Abdominal distension and blood in stools were seen. Pneumatosis intestinalis is a radiographic sign.

Qn. 134 Answer is b.

This scenario is typical of diaphragmatic hernia when increased distension of stomach leads to further compromise in the lung expansion due to herniated viscera to thorax.

Pediatrics e-MCQ

Qn.135 Answer is d.

Congenital CMV infection shows microcephaly and intraventricular calcifications, which have a predilection to CSF spaces. Intra parenchymal calcifications are seen in toxoplasmosis also. Rubella can cause thrombocytopenia

Qn. 136 Answer is a.

There is high incidence of leukemia in Down's syndrome. However the scenario presented is more likely a Leukemoid reaction

Qn. 137 Answer is a.

Infants born to mothers with diabetes can have various cardiac abnormalities including cardiomyopathy and VSD. Ebstein anomaly is not characteristically seen

Qn.138 Answer is e.

The following are the contraindications for using Indomethacin: Necrotizing entero colitis, gastro intestinal bleeding, Sepsis and Creatinine level more than 1.7mg/dL

Qn.139 Answer is c.

Pyruvate kinase deficiency is commonly seen as causing hyperbilirubinemia in infants of certain ethnic origin. This is due to hemolysis.

Qn.140 Answer is a.

The transplacental transfer of glucose cause islet cell hyperplasia in infant and thereby causing hyper insulinism and hypoglycemia.

Qn.141 Answer is e.

Pediatrics e-MCQ

Naloxone is used for respiratory depression due to narcotic. It is not used for opiate withdrawal.

Qn.142 Answer is b.

Fetal hemoglobin is resistant to alkali denaturation, whereas adult hemoglobin is susceptible to such denaturation. Therefore, exposing the blood specimen to sodium hydroxide will denature the adult but not the fetal hemoglobin. This is the basis for Apt test. The fetal hemoglobin will appear as a pinkish color under the microscope while the adult hemoglobin will appear as a yellow-brownish color. Swallowed maternal blood versus infant's blood can be assessed.

Kleihauer Betke test is used to quantitatively assess feto maternal hemorrhage, by detecting fetal blood in maternal circulation.

Qn.143 Answer is b.

Hypomagnesemia is seen in infants born to diabetic mothers which can lead to seizures

13. Nephrology

Qn.144 Answer is d.

Henoch Schonlein purpura can present with purpuric spots, arthritis, renal involvement and hypertension. Post streptococcal glomerulonephritis cause oliguria, hematuria. The purpura is not seen in Lupus and polyarteritis nodosa, even though renal involvement is seen. Meningococcemia has hemorrhagic rash and fever, which will be critical within hours.

Qn.145 Answer is b.

Hemolytic uremic syndrome often follow infection due to certain strains of E Coli.

This is characterized by intra vascular hemolysis and can be detected in the peripheral smear as fragmented RBCs and Schistocytes.

Qn.146 Answer is c.

An asymptomatic recurrent painless hematuria after respiratory infections is seen in IgA nephropathy. As there is no evidence of acute nephritis, post streptococcal glomerulonephritis is not present.

Qn. 147 Answer is d.

Acute post streptococcal glomerulonephritis presents as this classic features as described in the vignette. Hypertension leading to hypertensive encephalopathy is the reason for seizures. BP control is the definitive treatment for the encephalopathy.

Qn. 148 Answer is a.

Posterior urethral valves cause obstruction of urine flow leading to hydronephrosis.

Pediatrics e-MCQ

Qn. 149 Answer is d.

Chronically scarred kidneys resulting from vesico ureteric reflux and pyelonephritis can be the cause of hypertension in many adolescents.

Qn. 150 Answer is a.

Minimal change nephrotic syndrome produce massive edema and can present acutely. Usually the urine shows massive proteinuria without any red cell casts.

Qn. 151 Answer is c.

Amphotericin therapy leads to hypokalemia in some newborns.

Qn. 152 Answer is e.

Pediatrics e-MCQ

Renal tubular acidosis Distal type can present with this clinical picture

Qn.153 Answer is a.

Vesico ureteric reflux with additional left uretero pelvic junction obstruction causes the reduced outflow from the left kidney.

14. Neurology

Qn.154 Answer is d.

Benign Rolandic Epilepsy (Benign Epilepsy with Central Temporal Spikes) is the common cause of secondary generalized seizures in the age group of 4 years to 10 years. Many children have nocturnal seizures and majority are seizure free by puberty. Juvenile myoclonic epilepsy starts later in adolescence and have generalized poly spike and wave discharges in the EEG. Absence epilepsy can be associated with absence seizures as well as generalized tonic clonic seizures. EEG will show generalized 3 Hz spike and wave discharges. Central pontine myelinolysis is a condition related to rapid correction of hyponatremia, which will be associated with acute onset neurological deficit, not seizures. Febrile seizures do not have any evidence of epileptiform activity in EEG

Qn.155 Answer is d.

Acquired epileptiform aphasia (Landau Kleffner Syndrome) is a condition in which the patient who has normal speech

Pediatrics e-MCQ

development gets speech deficits due to ongoing seizures. This is rare.

There are no focal deficits to support a diagnosis of cerebral infarction. Mesial temporal sclerosis is a common structural etiology for complex partial seizures in adults. Some investigators hypothesized that mesial temporal sclerosis may be related to high seizure burden in childhood, like prolonged febrile seizures. However this is not a cause of speech deficits.

Qn.156 Answer is e.

Sudden onset paraplegia and absent reflexes suggest Guillain Barre syndrome, an ascending polyneuropathy. This can follow immunizations and infections like Campylobacter. Hypokalemic paralysis is usually temporary and brought about by exercise, high carbohydrate load etc. in patients with strong family history of periodic paralysis. Central pontine myelinolysis can produce a weakness, however reflexes may be present. Paralytic polio myelitis is rare and not seen in immunized children and usually encephalopathy or fever may be present. Transverse myelitis will present with sensory and motor deficits. Pain, a horizontal band of anesthesia or sensory level is usually seen.

Pediatrics e-MCQ

Qn. 157 Answer is e.

Neuroblastoma can cause ataxia, unusual chaotic eye movements and torticollis.

Urinary excretion of catecholamine metabolites can be characteristic finding.

There can be escalation of motor and vocal tics in children with ADHD treated with stimulant medications. However a thorough neurological examination can identify other neurological disorders coexisting in those children.

Qn. 158 Answer is c.

Infantile spasms usually get diagnosed only after 3-4 months of their initial presentation in infants. This is due to the lack of awareness among physicians and care takers and not recognizing the typical clinical presentation. The seizures occur as brief sudden flexion of neck and extremities, or extension of extremities lasting a second, repeated in clusters. Infantile spasms are difficult to treat, as commonly used anti-seizure medications are not successful. However, many children respond to ACTH treatment. Even though it is treatable, this carries high risk for neuro developmental disabilities in affected children.

Pediatrics e-MCQ

Qn. 159 Answer is b.

One of the commonest identifiable etiologies for infantile spasms is tuberous sclerosis. Patient's with tuberous sclerosis are also susceptible to other seizures later in their life.

Qn. 160 Answer is d.

A boy with proximal muscle weakness as characterized by inability to stand up from sitting position and waddling gait should arouse suspicion of muscle disease. Absence of dermatological findings (like rash, papules over fingers) makes it less likely to be juvenile dermatomyositis. Duchenne muscular dystrophy is likely in this case even though reflexes are present.

Qn. 161 Answer is b.

Roseola is a viral infection most commonly produce high fevers and also commonly cause febrile seizures in genetically susceptible children.

Pediatrics e-MCQ

Absence of encephalopathy and signs of meningeal irritation makes it less likely to be meningitis. Kawasaki syndrome usually presents with fever for many days and desquamating rash, mucosal involvement and swelling of hands and feet.

Qn. 162 Answer is a.

Childhood absence epilepsy is manifested by abrupt onset unresponsiveness and loss of consciousness lasting for 10-20 seconds, sometimes associated with eye lid fluttering and then rapid return to baseline without confusion or drowsiness. Hyper ventilation can trigger a seizure.

Qn.163 Answer is d.

Sturge Weber syndrome with port wine stain can also have intracranial / leptomeningeal angiomatosis. Affected individuals are prone to seizures

The distribution of the hemangioma is mostly over the face, scalp and neck region.

Qn.164 Answer is b.

Pediatrics e-MCQ

Acute cerebellar ataxia is a diagnosis by exclusion of conditions as mentioned.

This entity is usually post infectious and self-limited, but with sometimes significant gait issues will develop, which can last for few days.

Qn.165 Answer is a.

Sleep terrors or night terrors cause significant anxiety in parents. Children are awakened by fear and can continue inconsolable crying for up to 30 minutes. This is an age related phenomenon and will resolve spontaneously. This has no connection with epilepsy or other organic causes. There are no tonic clonic activity or staring noticed with these events. Work up is not necessary

Qn.166 Answer is e.

Facial weakness due to bilateral lower motor neuron facial palsy can cause inability to close eyes. Myasthenia can cause droopy eyes, but there will be wrinkles over the forehead. Psychogenic blepharospasm can sometimes be a problem in patients with conversion disorder. Lead encephalopathy does not present like this.

Qn.167 Answer is a.

Early fusion of cranial sutures (cranio synostosis) can cause microcephaly. This will have a restrictive effect on the brain growth. Rarely children will have signs of raised intracranial pressure. Dandy walker malformation cause cerebellar vermian hypoplasia and rarely cause hydrocephalus. Hyperthyroidism does not cause microcephaly.

Qn.168 Answer is c.

Erb's palsy or brachial plexus palsy can be seen in infants with history of shoulder dystocia. As there was no tenderness or crepitus in the clavicular area, fracture of clavicle is ruled out. Cerebral infarctions can be present in infants, but will not present at birth with focal deficits like this. Usually the upper extremity will be in a flexed position if that is present.

Pediatrics e-MCQ

15. Nutrition and Fluid Management

Qn.169 Answer is c.

Vitamin D deficiency is common in breast fed African American infants. The vignette describes an infant with features of Rickets. Elevated alkaline phosphatase is seen in these infants.

Qn. 170 Answer is a.

Vitamin A toxicity is manifested as intra cranial hypertension (pseudo tumor cerebri.) Nutritional supplements contain more than the daily requirements of vitamins. This can lead to toxicity or hyper Vitaminosis of lipid soluble vitamins.

Qn. 171 Answer is c.

Pyridoxine dependent seizures and pyridoxine deficiency seizures can manifest in the newborn period as refractory seizures.

Pediatrics e-MCQ

Qn. 172 Answer is a.

This infant should have alkaline phosphatase checked to rule out Vitamin D deficiency and Rickets

Qn. 173 Answer is a.

Prolonged total parenteral nutrition can cause various abnormalities and the commonest long term complication is cholestatic jaundice.

Adrenoleukodystrophy is characterized by elevated very long chain fatty acid levels in blood. Treatment involving medium chain and short chain fatty acids was used, but this has no relationship with total parenteral nutrition.

Pediatrics e-MCQ

16. Pediatric Surgery & orthopedics

Qn.174 Answer is d.

A subluxated radial head ("Nursemaid's Elbow") is a common injury in this age group with traction of elbow. This will cause acute pain and inability of movement of the elbow. Most of the time, during manipulation for radiographs, this will get corrected.

Fractures are common after falls.

Qn. 175 Answer is e.

This is typical of the Osgood Schlatter's disease or apophyseal traction and epiphysitis of the tibial tubercle. This is common in children who are active in sports. This causes pain and bony prominence below the knee. This will get resolved without any treatment.

Qn. 176 Answer is e.

Pediatrics e-MCQ

Anterior and posterior draw tests will evaluate the integrity of cruciate ligaments. As there is no locking on rotation, injuries of meniscus is unlikely. The tenderness over the lateral aspect points towards lateral collateral ligament injury

Qn. 177 Answer is c.

A negative wrist radiograph will not rule out injuries to metacarpal bones especially of the Scaphoid bone. The tenderness elicited in the anatomical snuff box area points towards fracture in this region.

Qn. 178 Answer is a.

A small bowel obstruction pattern as evidenced by multiple air fluid levels in this child with red stools is suggestive of intussusception, acute abdominal emergency. The cause of intussusception can be lymphoid hyperplasia in the small intestine secondary to infections. A barium enema can reduce the intussusception and can be both diagnostic and therapeutic.

Pediatrics e-MCQ

A delay in definitive treatment can be life threatening as it can cause bowel infarction and necrosis. Technetium scan is used to diagnose Meckel's diverticulitis.

Qn. 179 Answer is e.

This child has no evidence of infection, and no signs suggestive of formula intolerance. Meckel's diverticulum could be a one of the reasons for blood in stools and can be diagnosed by Meckel's scan.

Qn. 180 Answer is b.

Infection with Yersinia entero colitica can produce lower quadrant abdominal pain mimicking acute appendicitis.

Qn. 181 Answer is a.

Congenital diaphragmatic hernia commonly seen at left posterolateral location

Qn. 182 Answer is b.

Legg-Calve-Perthes disease usually occurs in boys 4 - 10 years old. There are many theories about the cause of this disease. Avascular necrosis of head of femur causing collapse and flattening of the head. Usually it is unilateral, but can be bilateral also.

Qn.183 Answer is b.

Teenage boys with obesity are prone to slipped capital femoral epiphysis.

This should be surgically fixed.

Qn.184 Answer is c.

Pediatrics e-MCQ

Six week old infant with increased hunger and projectile non bilious vomiting is possibly manifesting features of congenital hypertrophic pyloric stenosis.

Alkalosis and mild jaundice is sometimes seen.

Qn.185 Answer is a.

An elevated fat pad sign is pathognomonic for intra articular fracture of the humerus. He needs to be seen by an orthopedic specialist for plaster casting and hospitalization for observation for any neuro vascular injury.

Qn.186 Answer is b.

A blindly ending esophagus with respiratory distress on feeding is suggestive of trachea esophageal fistula and esophageal atresia. Infants with poor swallowing will often found to have history of polyhydramnios

Qn.187 Answer is d.

This pattern is suggestive of midgut volvulus and not typical of pyloric stenosis or duodenal atresia.

Qn.188 Answer is c.

Children with Downs syndrome are prone to develop duodenal atresia and the appearance of "double bubble" is characteristic.

Qn.189 Answer is d.

Delayed passage of meconium and meconium ileus is seen in cystic fibrosis. However dilated proximal bowel and narrow distal colon is suggestive of

Aganglionic segment as seen in Hirschsprung's disease.

Qn.190 Answer is e.

An undescended intra-abdominal testes can be subject to malignant transformation and needs to be removed. If it is retractile, there is a risk for injury and torsion and should have the orchiopexy.

Qn.191 Answer is b.

Cleft lip is corrected early and cleft palate at later stage. Cleft lip and cleft palate are due to multifactorial inheritance. Trisomy 18 is associated with cleft lip and palate and infants with these problems should also be screened for associated malformations.

17. Pulmonology

Qn.192 Answer is b.

Laryngomalacia is associated with inspiratory stridor, gastro esophageal reflux is commonly seen in children with floppy larynx and hypotonia. Pulmonary sequestration can cause infections and wheezing

Laryngotracheobronchitis(croup) is usually related to viral infections

Qn.193 Answer is e.

Immuno deficiencies including immunoglobulin subclass deficiencies and tests for cystic fibrosis may be indicated in the work up of recurrent infections. Anti neutrophil cytoplasmic antibodies are seen in vasculitides including Wegener's granulomatosis and Churg Strauss syndrome which are not indicated in the work up for etiologies of recurrent pulmonary infections.

Pediatrics e-MCQ

Qn. 194 Answer is d.

The other medications in the management of status asthmaticus include: Ketamine, Halothane, Magnesium sulfate and Ipratropium bromide. Nitric oxide is not used for this indication.

Qn. 195 Answer is a.

Airway hyper reactivity in children can be diagnosed using Methacholine challenge. Helium oxygen mixture is used in treatment of severe asthma.

Pilocarpine and atropine are also not used for this purpose

Qn. 196 Answer is b.

Decreased breath sounds associated with ipsilateral tracheal deviation in this patient point towards atelectasis, which was noted in the chest x-ray. The common problem of mucus plugging the airways can cause atelectasis

Pediatrics e-MCQ

Qn. 197 Answer is c.

Complete choanal atresia is not an uncommon problem in newborns. As newborns are obligatory mouth breathers, as soon as they get obstruction of nasal passages, they end up having respiratory distress, Inability to pass a nasal cannula can give clue to diagnosis.

Pediatrics e-MCQ

18. Rheumatology

Qn.198 Answer is d.

Factor VIII deficiency can present with purpura.

Qn. 199 Answer is c.

Juvenile rheumatoid arthritis can develop splenomegaly, leukopenia and rash.

Qn. 200 Answer is e.

Juvenile dermatomyositis is the commonest inflammatory myopathy of children.

Apart from a violaceous malar rash, they have nail fold telangiectasia

Pediatrics e-MCQ

Qn. 201 Answer is c.

SLE characteristically shows low Complement (C3 and C4) levels

Qn. 202 Answer is d.

Children with uveitis are commonly ANA positive

/END/

Pediatrics e-MCQ

Pediatrics e-MCQ

We are all in the gutter, but some of us are looking at the stars.

Oscar Wilde

www.ingramcontent.com/pod-product-compliance
Lightning Source LLC
Chambersburg PA
CBHW061503180526
45171CB00001B/25